D0128981

FIRST AID
FAST
for
Babies
and Children

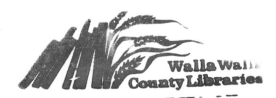

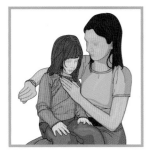
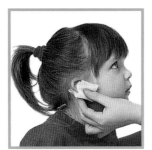
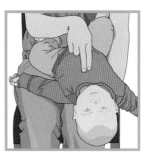
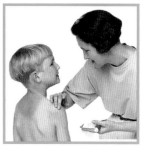

FIRST AID
FAST
for
Babies
and Children

Emergency procedures for all parents and caregivers

Medical Editor

Dr. Gina M. Piazza, FACEP

Penguin
Random
House

DK LONDON
Consultant Editor Jemima Dunne
Senior Art Editor Sharon Spencer
Project Editor Miezan van Zyl
Jacket Designer Mark Cavanagh
Managing Editor Angeles Gavira
Managing Art Editor Michael Duffy
Pre-Production Producer Andy Hilliard
Producer Jude Crozier
Art Director Karen Self
Publisher Liz Wheeler
Publishing Director Jonathan Metcalf

DK INDIA
Art Editors Konica Juneja, Anjali Sachar
Senior DTP Designers Vishal Bhatia, Sachin Singh
Managing Editor Rohan Sinha
Deputy Managing Art Editor Anjana Nair
Pre-production Manager Balwant Singh
Production Manager Pankaj Sharma
Jacket Designer Dhirendra Singh
Managing Jackets Editor Sreshtha Bhattacharya

DK US
US Editors Jill Hamilton, Dr. Gina Piazza, Lori Hand

First American Edition, 1994
This edition published in the United States in 2017 by DK Publishing,
345 Hudson Street, New York, New York 10014

A catalog record for this book is available from the Library of Congress.
ISBN 978-1-4654-5952-7

DK books are available at special discounts when purchased
in bulk for sales promotions, premiums, fund-raising, or
educational use. For details, contact: DK Publishing Special
Markets, 345 Hudson Street, New York, New York 10014
SpecialSales@dk.com

Printed and bound in China

All images © Dorling Kindersley Limited
For further information see: www.dkimages.com

A WORLD OF IDEAS:
SEE ALL THERE IS TO KNOW
www.dk.com

Disclaimer:
First Aid Fast for Babies and Children provides information and guidance on initial care following an incident or if
a child is unwell, but should not be regarded as a substitute for medical advice. The publisher and medical editor
do not accept responsibility for any claims arising from the use of this manual.

Foreword

Being a parent, grandparent, or caregiver to a child can be extraordinarily rewarding, but it can also be terrifying if a child in your care becomes ill or injured. If that were to happen, would you know what to do? Do you have the skills to render immediate lifesaving aid? Do you know how to access advanced care to help you rescue an ill or injured child? Are you prepared to act if the need arises?

Children are curious, and as they set out to learn they may endure injuries—from minor cuts, scrapes, and bruises to more serious injuries like fractured bones or head injuries. And, as children grow and are exposed to the environment and people around them, they will undoubtedly contract a variety of illnesses. When illness or injury strikes, should you call 911, visit the doctor, or simply provide care at home? This revised edition of *First Aid Fast for Babies and Children* can help you learn how to respond appropriately to a variety of injuries and illnesses. It contains the latest guidelines for lifesaving emergency care laid out in an easy-to-follow format.

After reading this book, I hope you will feel more confident in your ability to provide immediate care when a child falls ill or is injured while in your presence. Keep it handy and refer to it if you if have a question about how to correctly render aid in a given circumstance. You have the ability to reduce suffering and to save a life.

Dr. Gina M. Piazza, FACEP

Contents

Introduction 8

How to use this book 9

Action in an
Emergency 10
Fire 11
Electrical injury 12
Water incident 13
Checking vital signs 14

Unresponsiveness 16
Unresponsiveness 16
Unresponsive baby 19
CPR: baby 20
Unresponsive child 22
CPR: child 24
Recovery position 26

Breathing Difficulties 28
Choking baby 28
Choking child 30
Breath holding 32
Hiccups 32

Suffocation and
strangulation 33
Fume inhalation 33
Croup 34
Asthma 35

Wounds and Bleeding 36
Shock 36
Severe bleeding 38
Embedded object 40
Cuts and abrasions 41
Infected wound 42
Blisters 43
Eyebrow or eyelid wounds 44
Nosebleed 45
Ear wound 46
Mouth wound 47
Amputation 48
Internal bleeding 49

Crush injury 49
Chest wound 50
Abdominal wound 51

Burns and Scalds 52
Burns and scalds 52
Electrical burn 54
Chemical burn to skin 55
Chemical burn to eye 56

Poisoning 57
Swallowed chemicals 57
Drug or alcohol poisoning 58
Plant poisoning 58

Head, Face, and
Spine Injuries 59
Scalp wound 59
Head injury 60
Nose or cheekbone injury 62
Jaw injury 62
Spine injury 63

Bone, Joint, and
Muscle Injuries 64
Pelvic injury 64
Leg injury 64
Knee injury 66
Foot injury 66
Ankle injury 67
Collarbone injury 68
Rib injury 69
Arm injury 70
Elbow injury 70

Hand injury 71
Finger injury 72
Cramp 73
Bruises and swelling 74

Foreign Objects 75
Splinter 75
Object in eye 76
Object in ear 77
Object in nose 78
Swallowed object 78

Bites and Stings 79
Animal and human bites 79
Insect sting 80
Poison ivy rash 80
Tick bite 81
Jellyfish sting 82
Marine puncture wound 82
Snakebite 83

Effects of Heat and Cold 84
Hypothermia 84
Frostbite 86
Sunburn 87
Heat rash 87
Heat exhaustion 88
Heatstroke 89

Medical Disorders 90
Allergy 90
Anaphylactic shock 91

Diabetic emergency 92
Fainting 93
Fever 94
Meningitis 95
Febrile seizures 96
Epileptic seizures 97
Vomiting and diarrhea 98
Stomachache 99
Earache 100
Toothache 101

First Aid Kit 102
First aid kit 102
Dressings 104
Bandaging 105
Triangular bandages 106
Useful household items 108

Home Safety 109
Safety at home 109
Hall and stairs 110
Living Room or
Family Room 111
Kitchen 112
Bedrooms 114
Bathroom 116
Toys and playthings 117
Yard 118

Garage and car safety 119
Out and about 120
Traveling with children 122

Index 123
Acknowledgments 127

Useful Telephone Numbers 128

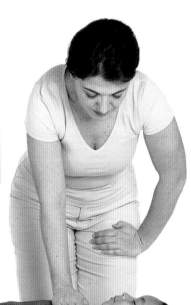

Introduction

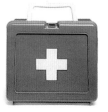

This book has been compiled primarily for parents but also for others—grandparents, teachers, playgroup leaders, and babysitters—who may regularly, or even just occasionally, find themselves in charge of babies and children. The content has been set out in a clear and logical way and the information is presented largely in pictorial form using simple words and captions to make it very easy to follow and to understand. The first aid advice given can be used to treat any age child and follows the most up-to-date clinical guidance at the time of publication.

Emergencies are, by their very nature, unexpected events and can be extremely frightening and stressful for anyone caring for a child. *First Aid Fast for Babies and Children* will help you learn various practical skills that will help you manage a wide range of first aid emergencies and everyday incidents, building your confidence and ensuring that you respond in the best way possible. The calmer you are, the more effective your help will be, and by listening and talking to the child you will be able to make the best decision for both of you, greatly improving the outcome.

In addition, there is reference information at the back of the book. A section on first aid kits and bandaging techniques also lists useful items to have at home and how to use them. The pages on Home Safety highlight potential danger areas around the home and how to fix them to minimize the risk of incidents in the first place.

How to use this book

This book covers first aid treatment for everything from minor cuts and abrasions to treating a child who is not responding. For every condition a series of photographs or illustrations shows you exactly what to do in an emergency. Key pieces of information are indicated on the photographs, and supplementary advice can be found alongside in the step-by-step text.

The injuries are organized by type, in colored sections such as Breathing Difficulties or Wounds and Bleeding. However, in an emergency, the thumbnail index on the back cover will direct you straight to the relevant page. There are also sections, such as Action in an Emergency, Bandages and Dressings, and Home Safety, that contain information for general reference.

Key signs and symptoms help you recognize the conditions

Annotations highlight essential action

Clear photographs illustrate every step of treatment

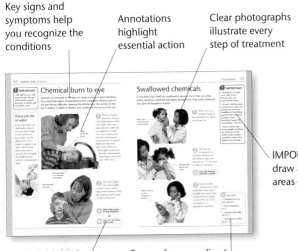

IMPORTANT boxes draw attention to areas of concern

Symbols highlight the action necessary for medical help

Cross references direct you to pages with information about associated injuries

Guide to the symbols

The following symbols and instructions appear if your child needs further medical attention:

 SEEK MEDICAL ADVICE

Depending on your area, call your doctor's office, nurse practitioner, or on-call service for advice.

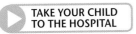 **TAKE YOUR CHILD TO THE HOSPITAL**

Take your child to the nearest hospital emergency department if you have help and transportation.

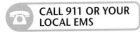 **CALL 911 OR YOUR LOCAL EMS**

Your child needs urgent medical attention and is best transported by trained medical experts to the hospital.

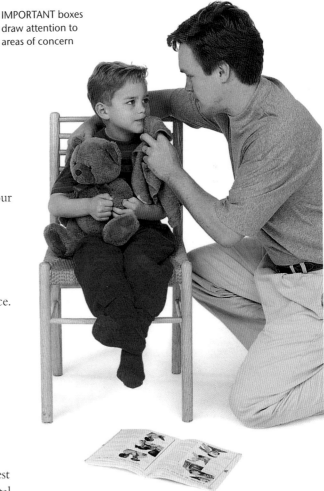

Action in an emergency

In any emergency, particularly one involving children, it is important to remain calm and act logically. Remember four steps:

① Assess the situation

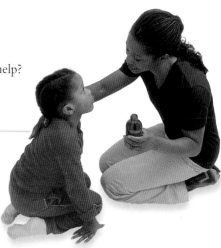

- What happened and how did it happen?
- Is it safe for you to approach?
- Is there more than one injured child?
- Is there anyone who can help?
- Do you need emergency medical services?

② Safety is important

- Do not risk injuring yourself—you cannot help if you become a casualty.
- Remove any source of danger from your child. Move your child only if it is safe for you and it's essential for her safety, and do so very carefully.

③ Treat serious injuries first

The primary considerations that immediately threaten life are:
- Serious bleeding, which can result in life-threatening shock (*see p. 36*).
- Obstructed airway, which prevents breathing, can result in the heart stopping (*see p. 16*).

> **! IMPORTANT**
> - **If more than one child is injured, go to the quiet one;** she may be unresponsive and not breathing.

④ Get help

Shout for help early and ask others to:
- Make the area safe.
- Seek medical advice or call 911.
- Help with first aid.
- Move a child to safety, if necessary.

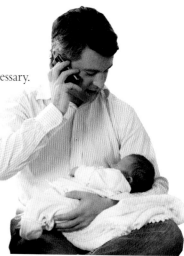

Telephoning for help

When you call 911 or your local EMS, use a hands-free phone so that you can treat the child at the same time. Provide the following:
- Your telephone number.
- The location of the incident.
- The type of incident.
- The number, sex, and ages of the casualties.
- Details of injuries.
- Information about hazards such as gas, power lines, or fog.

Fire

Write down an escape plan for your home and make sure everyone knows what to do.
- How would you get out of each room?
- How do you help babies and young children?
- Where will you meet when you've escaped?

Action for a frying pan fire

- Turn off heat source, then cover pan with lid, wet dishtowel, or fire blanket. Leave this on for half an hour—NEVER throw water over the flames.
- If fire is not under control, get out of the house, close doors behind you, and call the fire department.

Escaping from a fire

 Feel the door. If the door is cool, leave the room.

OR

 If the door is hot, don't open it. Go to the window.

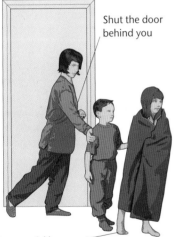

Shut the door behind you

Leave quickly
DO NOT GO BACK

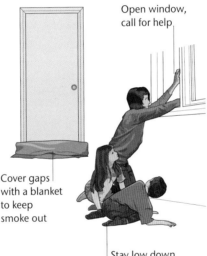

Open window, call for help

Cover gaps with a blanket to keep smoke out

Stay low down where air is clearest

⚠ IMPORTANT

- **Carry** babies and toddlers.
- **Don't** ask children to do anything other than look after themselves.
- **Close** all doors behind you.
- **Meet** outside your house.
- **Never** go back inside.
- **Phone** for help from elsewhere.

If you have to escape through a window:
- **If** you have to break the glass, put a blanket over the frame before you escape.
- **Slide** your child out, hang onto him, then ask him to drop down, if it is safe to do so.
- **Slide** out yourself, hang from the ledge, then drop.

Clothing on fire

If clothing is on fire:
Stop your child from moving; movement will fan the flames.
Drop him to the floor and wrap him in a coat or blanket, if available, to help smother the flames.
Roll him on the ground.

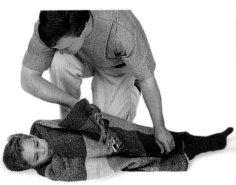

⚠ IMPORTANT

- **Do not** let your child run around; rapid movement will fan the flames.
- **If** water is available, lay him down, burning side uppermost, and douse him with water or a nonflammable liquid.

Electrical injury

Children are at risk of injury from domestic electricity if they play with electrical sockets or cords, or if cords are worn. Electrical current causes muscle spasms that keep a child from letting go of an electric cord and may cause burns both where the current enters and where it leaves the child's body. The current may also cause breathing and heart to stop.

High-voltage current

Contact with electricity from power lines and overhead cables is usually fatal. Severe burns result and the child may be thrown some distance from the point of contact. DO NOT approach the child unless you are officially informed that the power has been cut off.

see also

● Checking vital signs, p.14

● Electrical burn, p.54

● Unresponsive baby, pp.19–21

● Unresponsive child, pp.22–27

☎ **CALL 911 OR YOUR LOCAL EMS**

1 Do not touch the child. Break the contact with electricity by turning the current off at the main switch.

2 If you cannot turn off the current, stand on dry insulating material such as large paperback books or a wooden box. Use a wooden broom handle or chair to separate your child's limbs from the source.

Stand on insulating material

Use nonconducting object

Push the source away

3 If you still cannot break the contact without touching your child, wrap a dry towel or rubberized exercise band around his feet and pull him away from the source.

Wrap a dry towel around his feet

4 Once the contact is broken, treat any injuries. If the child appears unharmed, monitor his breathing, pulse, and response while waiting for help.

Water incident

Babies and young children can drown quickly if they slip into a pool or pond or are left unattended in a bath. Even 1in in a bath, or several inches in a bucket of water is enough to cover a baby's nose and mouth if he falls forward.

! IMPORTANT

● **Do not** put yourself in danger when attempting a rescue; don't enter the water unless you have to in order to save the child's life or you are a trained lifesaver.

● **If** the child is too small to follow commands, or unable, you may have to go in and rescue the child if possible.

● **Always** seek medical advice even if the child appears to have recovered because he may have inhaled some water, which can cause lung damage.

● **If** your child becomes unresponsive and is not breathing normally, begin CPR with 30 compressions immediately. CALL 911 OR YOUR LOCAL EMS.

● **Be** prepared to roll the child onto his side to clear airway because it is possible that he may regurgitate his stomach contents.

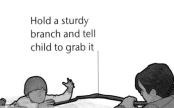

Hold a sturdy branch and tell child to grab it

Lie on bank so you don't fall in

1 Get the child out of the water as quickly as possible. If the child is conscious and able to follow directions, hold out a branch or rope for the child to grab, or throw him anything that will float.

2 Once the child is out of the water, protect him from cold and get him to a shelter. Treat him for hypothermia and replace any wet clothes with dry ones as soon as possible. Even if the child seems to have recovered,

Start warming child as soon as he is out of water

> ▶ **TAKE YOUR CHILD TO THE HOSPITAL**

OR

> ☎ **CALL 911 OR YOUR LOCAL EMS**

DROWNING CHAIN OF SURVIVAL FOR UNTRAINED RESCUER

Prevent drowning	Recognize distress	Provide flotation	Remove from water	Give first aid
Stay safe and supervise your child in and around water.	Ask someone to call for help if the child is in distress.	Getting a float to a child can prevent submersion.	Attempt this only if it is safe to do so.	Treat as appropriate and seek medical advice.

≫ see also

● Hypothermia, *p.84*

● Unresponsive baby, *pp.19–21*

● Unresponsive child, *pp.22–27*

Checking vital signs

When you are looking after a baby or child who is sick or injured, you need to check her vital signs—breathing, pulse, level of response, and fever—as part of assessing the severity of a condition. Then continue to monitor the signs while you are looking after your child or waiting for medical help to arrive, because the information can indicate whether a child's condition is changing (either improving or deteriorating). Note that here you are checking and monitoring for quality of pulse or breathing, not the presence or absence of them.

Breathing

When assessing breathing you are looking at how many times a child breathes in a minute, as well as the quality of the breaths—for example depth and ease. A baby may breathe as many as 40 breaths a minute; a toddler or child up to five years, 20–30 times; a child up to 12 years old, 12–25 times a minute; and an older child, about 12–18 breaths.

You can sit with the child and watch and listen for breaths, or for a baby or younger child it may be better to place your hand on the chest. Make a note of the breathing rate (the number of breaths in a minute) and as well as whether they are deep or shallow, easy or difficult, painful and/or quiet or noisy—and if the latter, what do they sound like?

Time the breaths with your watch

Check breathing Rate
Sit your child down or on your lap. Place one hand on her chest. Count the number of times she breathes in a minute and listen to the breaths.

Pulse

Every time the heart beats, a wave of pressure passes along the blood vessels that carry blood from the heart to the body (arteries). This "wave" can be felt where the arteries lie close to the skin. For a baby check the pulse in the upper arm; for older children check it at the wrist. The normal pulse rate for an infant is 100–140, but it decreases with age. A toddler has a heart rate of 85–130; at ages 2–5, 80–115; for 5–12-year-olds, 75–110; and over 12 years, 60–100. Count the rate (number of beats in a minute), and note whether it is strong or weak and regular or irregular.

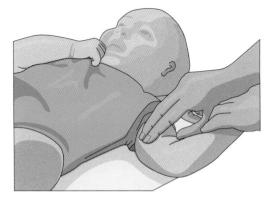

Use the pads of your fingers

BRACHIAL PULSE
Place the pads of two fingers against the inner side of the baby's upper arm.

RADIAL PULSE
Place the pads of two or three fingers on the forearm just below the wrist creases at the base of the thumb.

Level of response

Some illnesses and injuries can affect your child's level of response and she may be fully alert or totally unresponsive or somewhere between. Assess your child right away and then again at regular intervals.

• *Child is fully alert* Her eyes will be open and she responds normally when you ask questions.

• *Responds only to voice* Does your child answer simple questions and obey instructions? Can she open her eyes?

• *Responds only to pain* Does your child open her eyes or move if you tap her shoulder or flick her foot?

• *Unresponsive* The child does not respond to any stimulus.

Body Temperature

● Viral and bacterial infections, including colds, flu, bronchitis, and gastrointestinal and urinary tract infections, are the most common causes of a raised body temperature.

● A body temperature below 95°F (35°C) indicates hypothermia.

● The temperature that should be checked by a doctor increases with age. For infants under three months of age, seek medical advice for a fever of 100.4°F (38°C), measured rectally. In toddlers, a rectal temperature over 102.2°F (39°C) should be checked. In older children, a temperature over 103.3°F (39.6°C) should be investigated by a doctor.

● A child with a temperature above 104°F (40°C) is at risk of a febrile seizure.

Unresponsiveness

A baby or child needs to inhale oxygen into his lungs. This oxygen passes into the bloodstream and is pumped around the body by the heart. If a baby or child is unresponsive, the air passage, or airway, to the lungs may be blocked, which means oxygen can't enter the body. Lack of oxygen slows down the heartbeat until it stops altogether (cardiac arrest) and no oxygen will reach the brain.

What you can do to help

Always make sure it is safe to approach the baby or child; you can't help him if you become a casualty too. If you are certain you are safe, first assess whether he is responsive. If he is unresponsive and his breathing is abnormal or absent, you need to help pump some blood by doing chest compressions. If circulation stops, blood cannot travel around the body and vital organs such as the brain and heart are deprived of oxygen. Start CPR immediately with 30 chest compressions, followed by opening the airway so that you can breathe into the lungs. The combination of rescue breaths and chest compressions is known as cardiopulmonary resuscitation (CPR). An AED can be used to restore a normal heartbeat (*see p.23*).

Chain of survival

An unresponsive baby or child's chances of survival are greater if:
- You call for expert help;
- CPR is given as soon as possible;
- An AED is used early;
- Advanced care by healthcare professionals is received as soon as possible.

For a baby

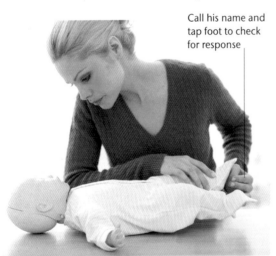

Call his name and tap foot to check for response

For a child

Call your child's name and tap shoulder to check for a response

When to call 911 or your local EMS

If there is somebody else present to help, always ask him or her to call 911 as soon as you realize that your child is not breathing. If you are on your own, give a combination of 30 chest compressions and 2 rescue breaths (CPR: baby *p.20*, child *p.24*) for two minutes before stopping to make the call. Then continue CPR until help arrives or the child recovers.

Maintain blood circulation

If your baby or child's heart has stopped beating, giving chest compressions will drive blood containing oxygen around the body. These will be more effective if alternated with rescue breaths. The combination of techniques is known as cardiopulmonary resuscitation (CPR).

For a child

For a baby

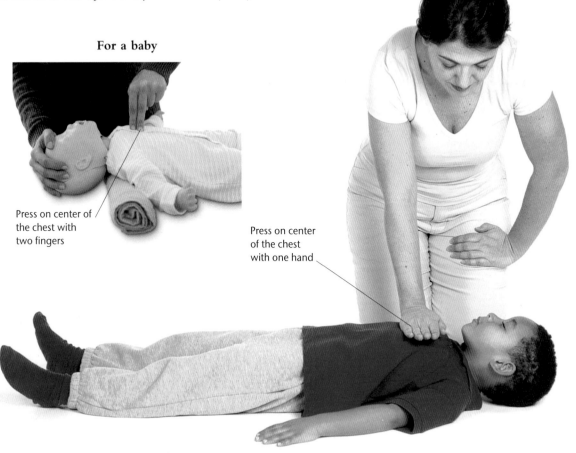

Press on center of the chest with two fingers

Press on center of the chest with one hand

Open the airway

You need to open the airway before you can give breaths. Place one hand on the forehead and gently tilt the head to bring the tongue away from the back of the throat. Place one or two fingers of your other hand on the chin to lift. If you suspect a neck injury, use the jaw thrust method to open the airway (see p.61).

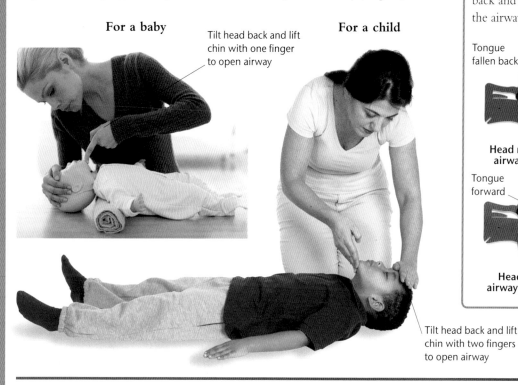

For a baby

Tilt head back and lift chin with one finger to open airway

For a child

Tilt head back and lift chin with two fingers to open airway

Airway

If a child is on his back the tongue may fall back and may block the airway.

Tongue fallen back

Head not tilted— airway blocked

Tongue forward

Head tilted— airway unblocked

Breathe for the baby or child

If your baby or child is not breathing, take a breath and blow oxygen into the child's lungs. This is known as rescue breathing.

For a child

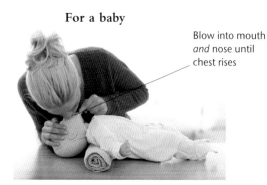

For a baby

Blow into mouth *and* nose until chest rises

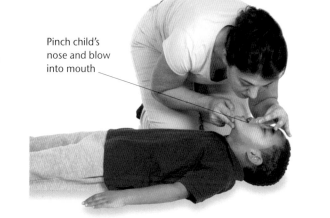

Pinch child's nose and blow into mouth

Unresponsive baby

Assess your baby before calling for help. If you are alone and the baby is not breathing, begin chest compressions and rescue breaths.

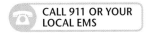 **Check for response**

- Call her name and tap her foot gently. Never shake a baby.
- If there is no response,

☎ **CALL 911 OR YOUR LOCAL EMS**

Tap foot

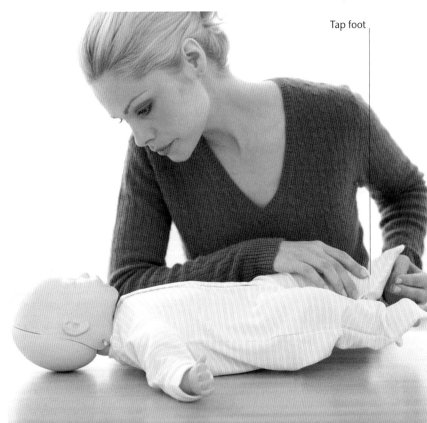

Resuscitation summary

Unresponsive baby

⬇

No breathing or just gasping

⬇

Send helper to

☎ **CALL 911 OR YOUR LOCAL EMS**

⬇

Start CPR: give 30 chest compressions

⬇

Open airway and give 2 rescue breaths

⬇

Repeat 30:2 for two minutes

⬇

If not already done,

☎ **CALL 911 OR YOUR LOCAL EMS**

⬇

Continue CPR until help arrives

! IMPORTANT
- **If** you are unable or unwilling to give rescue breaths, you can give chest compressions only.

Resuscitation summary

Unresponsive baby

⬇

No breathing or just gasping

⬇

Send helper to

📞 **CALL 911 OR YOUR LOCAL EMS**

⬇

Start CPR: give 30 chest compressions

⬇

Open airway and give 2 rescue breaths

⬇

Repeat 30:2 for two minutes

⬇

If not already done,

📞 **CALL 911 OR YOUR LOCAL EMS**

⬇

Continue CPR until help arrives

⚠ **IMPORTANT**

● **If** you are unable or unwilling to give rescue breaths, you can give chest compressions only.

CPR: baby

This is to be used for an unresponsive baby who is not breathing. Always start with 30 chest compressions, followed by two breaths. If you are alone, continue sets of 30 compressions and two breaths for two minutes before calling 911 or your local EMS.

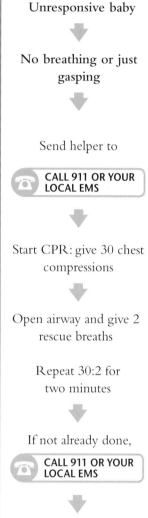

Press down by at least one-third of the depth of the chest

Place a towel roll under baby's shoulders

Lift point of chin with one finger

Tilt head back

Pick out visible obstructions

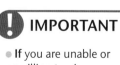

1 Begin chest compressions. Place two fingers of your lower hand on the center of the baby's chest. Press down vertically on the breastbone to depress it by at least one third of its depth. Release pressure, but don't move your fingers; allow the chest to come back up fully. Repeat to give 30 compressions at a rate of 100–120 per minute.

2 Make sure that her airway is open. Put your finger on the point of the chin and lift it. Take care not to press on the soft part of the neck under the chin because that can block the airway.

3 Pick out any visible obstruction from the mouth and nose with your fingertips.

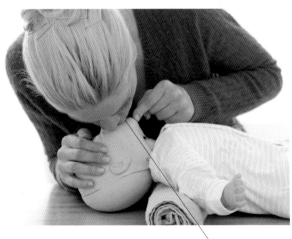

Repeat 30 chest compressions

Blow into the baby's mouth and nose

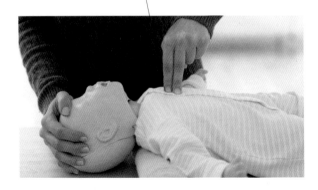

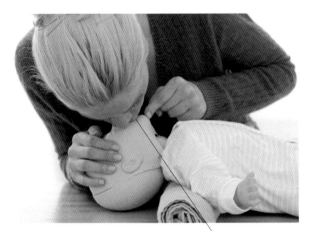

Follow with two rescue breaths

4 Take a normal breath, then seal your lips tightly around your baby's mouth and nose. Blow gently until you see the baby's chest rise—Do NOT blow the whole adult human breath into the baby. Do NOT remove mouth from baby's for this stage; just watch chest fall out of the corner of your eye.

5 Continue CPR with 30 chest compressions.

6 Return to the baby's head and give two rescue breaths, followed by another 30 chest compressions. Continue at a rate of 30:2 until the emergency services arrive; your baby shows signs of becoming responsive (coughing, opening her eyes, and moving) and she is breathing normally; or you are too exhausted to continue.

! IMPORTANT

● **Do not** sweep the mouth with your finger to search for an obstruction.

● **If** there is more than one rescuer, one gives 15 chest compressions followed by the other giving 2 breaths. There should be minimal pause between groups of compressions and breaths.

● **If** your baby shows signs of becoming responsive (*see left*) and she is breathing normally, cradle her in your arms with head tilted down until the ambulance arrives (*below*). Monitor breathing, pulse, and level of response (*see p.14*) until the help arrives.

The recovery position

Hold the baby in your arms with her head tilted downward and supported. This keeps her airway open and clear and allows fluid to drain away.

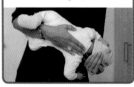

Resuscitation summary

Unresponsive child

⬇

No breathing or just gasping

⬇

Send helper to

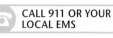
☎ **CALL 911 OR YOUR LOCAL EMS**

⬇

Start CPR: give 30 chest compressions followed by two rescue breaths

⬇

Repeat 30:2 for two minutes

⬇

If not already done,

☎ **CALL 911 OR YOUR LOCAL EMS**

⬇

Continue CPR until help arrives

⚠ **IMPORTANT**
● If you are unable or unwilling to give rescue breaths, you can give chest compressions only.

Unresponsive child

Assess a child (aged one year to puberty) before you call for help. If you are on your own and the child is not breathing or just gasping, begin CPR.

① Check for response

● Call his name, or tap his shoulder gently. Never shake a child.
● If there is no response,

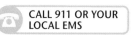
☎ **CALL 911 OR YOUR LOCAL EMS**

Tap his shoulder gently

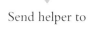

Using an AED on a child

Machines called AEDs can be used to analyze the heart rhythm and if necessary correct it by delivering an electric shock. If a child is unresponsive and not breathing, start chest compressions, followed by rescue breaths (CPR, *see p.24*), CALL 911 OR YOUR LOCAL EMS. Ask a helper to find an AED and use it as soon as it arrives—don't leave the child to look for one yourself. The machine will give you audible prompts to follow. If a shock is needed, the machine will deliver it; if not, it will not be given.

1 Turn on the machine. Pads may be connected to the machine (if not, the machine will tell you to connect them). If there are both adult and pediatric pads in the kit, use the right ones for the child's size.

2 Place the pads directly onto the child's chest. Peel off the backing paper and put one on the upper right side of the child's chest and the other on her lower left side.

3 Once the pads are attached, make sure no one is touching the child. The AED will analyze the heart rhythm and may recommend delivering a shock. Listen to the machine's instructions.

IF A SHOCK IS ADVISED
- The AED will start to charge up—make sure everyone is clear of the child, then follow the machine's prompts to deliver the shock.
- Continue CPR for 2 minutes or until the machine asks you to stop.
- The AED will reanalyze the child's heart rhythm at regular intervals; listen to the prompts.

IF A SHOCK IS NOT ADVISED
- Continue CPR. The AED will reanalyze the child's heart rhythm at regular intervals.

Ask all helpers to stay clear of the child during analysis and shock

Place one pad on left side of chest so that long axis is vertical

AED

Place one pad on upper right side of chest

! IMPORTANT

- **If** there are both adult and pediatric pads in the AED, use the pediatric ones, but adult pads can be used if pediatric pads are not available.

- **If** the child is very small, place one pad in the center of her back and the other one in the center of the chest. Both pads should be vertical.

- **If** she starts coughing, opening her eyes, speaking or moving purposefully, and is breathing normally, leave pads attached and put her in the recovery position.

Resuscitation summary

Unresponsive child

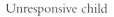

No breathing or just gasping

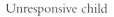

Send helper to

☎ **CALL 911 OR YOUR LOCAL EMS**

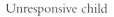

Start CPR: give 30 chest compressions, followed by two rescue breaths

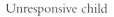

Repeat 30:2 for two minutes

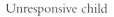

If not already done,

☎ **CALL 911 OR YOUR LOCAL EMS**

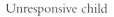

Continue CPR until help arrives

❗ **IMPORTANT**
● If you are unable or unwilling to give rescue breaths, you can give chest compressions only.

CPR: child

This is to be used for an unresponsive child who is not breathing. Always start with 30 chest compressions, followed by two breaths. If on your own, give CPR for two minutes before calling 911 or your local EMS.

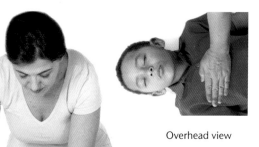

Overhead view

Press down by at least one-third of the depth of the chest

1 Begin chest compressions. Place the heel of one hand over the center of the child's chest (on the breastbone). Lean forward over the child so that your shoulder is directly above your hand. Press down vertically to depress the breastbone by at least one-third of its depth.

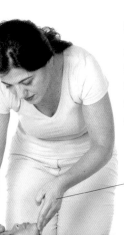

2 Release the pressure but don't move your hand; let the chest come back up. Repeat to give 30 compressions at a rate of 100–120 per minute.

Tilt head back

3 Make sure that the child's airway is open. Put your fingers on the point of the chin and lift it. Take care not to press on the soft part of the neck under the chin, because that can block the airway. Pick out any visible obstructions from the child's mouth with your fingertips.

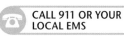

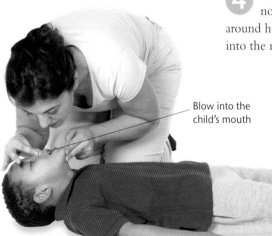

4 Pinch the child's nose. Take a normal breath, seal your lips around his mouth, and blow steadily into the mouth; the chest should rise.

Blow into the child's mouth

5 Remove your mouth, but not your hands, and watch the chest fall— this is a rescue breath. Each complete rescue breath should take one second.

6 Continue at a rate of 30:2 until the emergency services arrive; your child shows signs of becoming responsive (coughing, opening eyes, speaking, and moving purposefully) and is breathing normally; or you are too exhausted to continue.

! IMPORTANT

● **Do not** sweep mouth with your finger to search for an obstruction.

● **If** there is more than one rescuer, one gives 15 chest compressions followed by the other giving 2 breaths. There should be minimal pause between groups of compressions and breaths.

● **If** your child shows signs of becoming responsive (*see left*), and is breathing normally, place him in the recovery position (*see p.26*). Monitor breathing, pulse, and level of response (*see p.14*) until help arrives.

For a larger child or small rescuer

If the child is large or you are small, you can deliver chest compressions with two hands. Place the heel of one hand on the breastbone, in the center of the child's chest, then put your other hand on top and interlock your fingers. Then press down firmly to deliver compressions as above.

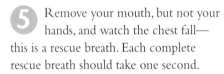

Interlock your fingers

Keep your fingers off the child's chest

Eyeglasses

If the child is wearing eyeglasses, remove them and keep them safe.

Recovery position

Put your child in this position if she is unresponsive but breathing to prevent her tongue or vomit from blocking her airway. If the child is found lying on her side or front, not all the steps will be needed.

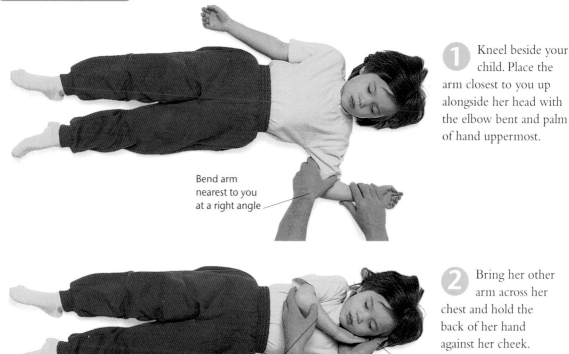

Bend arm nearest to you at a right angle

1 Kneel beside your child. Place the arm closest to you up alongside her head with the elbow bent and palm of hand uppermost.

Move farthest arm across her chest

Hold hand against her cheek

2 Bring her other arm across her chest and hold the back of her hand against her cheek.

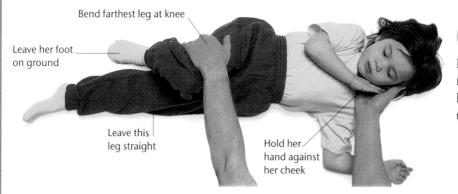

Bend farthest leg at knee

Leave her foot on ground

Leave this leg straight

Hold her hand against her cheek

3 With your other hand, pull up the knee of the leg farthest from you to bend the leg, leaving the foot on the ground.

4 Pull the bent leg toward you to roll your child onto her side. Keep your child's hand against her cheek to support her head.

Hold her hand against her cheek

Roll her over onto her side by pulling bent leg

5 Adjust her uppermost leg so she cannot fall forward, and tilt her head back to make sure her airway is open.

☎ **CALL 911 OR YOUR LOCAL EMS**

Tilt head back to make sure airway is still open

Keep lower leg straight

Bend top leg so that hips and knees form right angles to keep her from rolling forward

6 Check your child's breathing, pulse, and level of response while you are waiting for help to arrive.

>> *see also*
● Checking vital signs, *p.14*

Choking baby

If the baby has an incomplete airway obstruction, he may be coughing, have noisy breathing, or be in distress. If he is choking, there will be no noise. Give chest compressions then back blows to relieve a blockage.

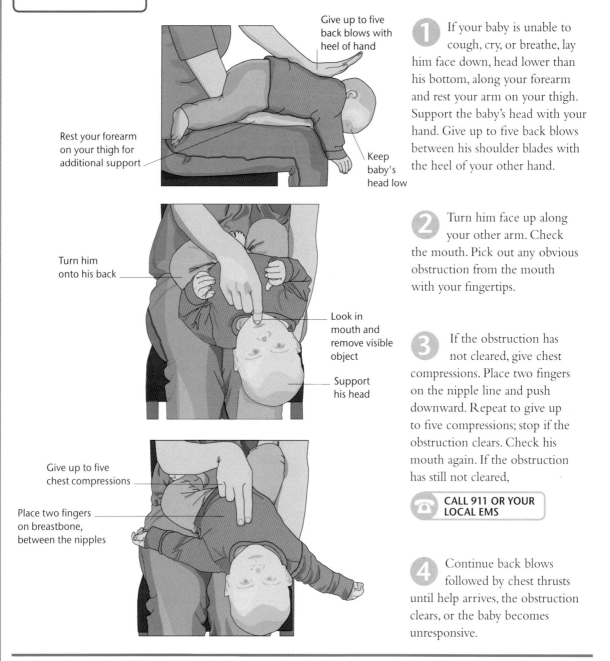

Give up to five back blows with heel of hand

Rest your forearm on your thigh for additional support

Keep baby's head low

Turn him onto his back

Look in mouth and remove visible object

Support his head

Give up to five chest compressions

Place two fingers on breastbone, between the nipples

1 If your baby is unable to cough, cry, or breathe, lay him face down, head lower than his bottom, along your forearm and rest your arm on your thigh. Support the baby's head with your hand. Give up to five back blows between his shoulder blades with the heel of your other hand.

2 Turn him face up along your other arm. Check the mouth. Pick out any obvious obstruction from the mouth with your fingertips.

3 If the obstruction has not cleared, give chest compressions. Place two fingers on the nipple line and push downward. Repeat to give up to five compressions; stop if the obstruction clears. Check his mouth again. If the obstruction has still not cleared,

☎ **CALL 911 OR YOUR LOCAL EMS**

4 Continue back blows followed by chest thrusts until help arrives, the obstruction clears, or the baby becomes unresponsive.

If your baby becomes unresponsive

If your choking baby becomes unresponsive, begin CPR. If he starts breathing at any stage, cradle him in your arms with his head down in the recovery position (*see p.21*).

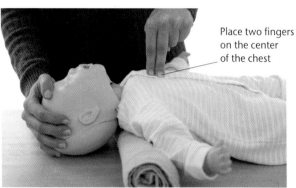

Place two fingers on the center of the chest

1 Give 30 chest compressions (this may dislodge obstruction).

2 If your baby is not breathing, clear any visible obstruction from his mouth; do not do a fingersweep.

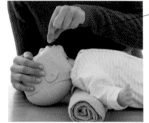

Remove visible obstructions

3 Begin rescue breaths. Give two rescue breaths by breathing into your baby's mouth and nose.

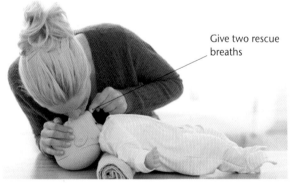

Give two rescue breaths

4 Repeat 30 chest compressions, then two rescue breaths. Continue to give 30 compressions followed by two rescue breaths for two minutes.

CALL 911 OR YOUR LOCAL EMS

Give 30 chest compressions

Follow with two breaths

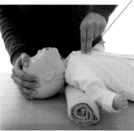

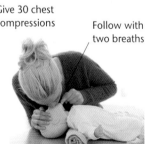

5 Continue alternating 30 chest compressions with two rescue breaths until help arrives, your baby shows signs of recovery (*see box, right*), or you are too exhausted to continue.

IMPORTANT

● **If** your baby shows signs of recovery such as coughing, opening his eyes, and moving purposefully, and is breathing normally, CALL 911 OR YOUR LOCAL EMS if not already done. Cradle him in your arms with head tilted down (recovery position) until emergency help arrives. Monitor breathing, pulse, and level of response until help arrives.

≫ *see also*

● Checking vital signs, *p.14*

● Unresponsive baby, *pp.19–21*

Choking child

Start by asking your child if she is choking. If the blockage is mild, she will be able to speak, cough, and breathe. If it is severe, she will not be able to speak, cough, or breathe.

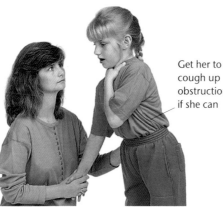

Get her to cough up obstruction if she can

1 If your child can cough, encourage her to do so to remove the object.

Press into her abdomen with quick upward thrusts

Stand behind her and wrap your arms around her waist

2 Stand or kneel behind her, and wrap your arms around her waist. Make a fist with one hand. Place the thumb side of your fist against the middle of her abdomen, just above her navel.

Press into her abdomen with quick upward thrusts

Grasp fist with your other hand

3 Grasp your fist with the other hand and press into her abdomen with a quick upward thrust.

4 Repeat step 3 until the obstruction clears or the child becomes unresponsive.

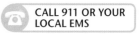
☎ **CALL 911 OR YOUR LOCAL EMS**

If your child becomes unresponsive

If your choking child becomes unresponsive, lower him to the floor, and treat as shown below. Send someone to CALL 911 OR YOUR LOCAL EMS.

Place one hand on center of the chest

Give 30 chest compressions

1 Begin CPR with 30 chest compressions (this may dislodge the obstruction).

Tilt head to open airway

2 Open his airway. If your child is not breathing, clear any visible obstruction from his mouth. Do not do a blind finger sweep.

Give two rescue breaths

3 Attempt two rescue breaths into the nose. Continue to give 30 compressions followed by two rescue breaths for 2 minutes.

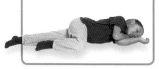 **CALL 911 OR YOUR LOCAL EMS**

Give 30 chest compressions

4 Continue cycles of 30 chest compressions followed by two rescue breaths until help arrives, your child resumes breathing, or you become too exhausted to continue.

The recovery position

If the child starts breathing again but remains unresponsive, place him in the recovery position and CALL 911 OR YOUR LOCAL EMS.

» *see also*
● Unresponsive child, *pp.22–29*

❗ IMPORTANT

● **Do not** shake a baby or young child.

● **If** he becomes unresponsive, open the airway and check breathing. If he is breathing, place him in the recovery position. CALL 911.

Breath holding

This is the result of rage and frustration. Your child is holding his breath if he cries, then breathes in but does not breathe out. He may go blue in the face and stiff and may even become unresponsive momentarily.

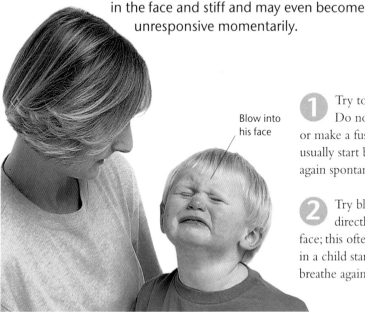

Blow into his face

1 Try to stay calm. Do not shake him or make a fuss. He will usually start breathing again spontaneously.

2 Try blowing directly into his face; this often results in a child starting to breathe again.

»» see also

● Unresponsive child, pp.22–27

❗ IMPORTANT

● **If** the hiccups go on for longer than a few hours, SEEK MEDICAL ADVICE. A long attack can be worrying, tiring, and painful.

Hiccups

These are very common and usually only last for a few minutes, but often seem to go on for a long time. Children can become distressed.

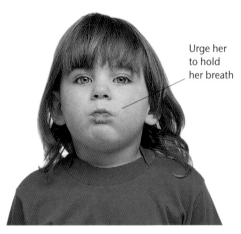

Urge her to hold her breath

1 Tell your child to sit still and hold her breath for 5–10 seconds, then encourage her to breathe out slowly.

2 Get her to repeat this until hiccups have stopped.

Suffocation and strangulation

Strangulation results from a constriction around the child's neck that prevents breathing. Suffocation occurs when there is an obstruction over the mouth or nose, a weight on the child's chest or abdomen preventing normal breathing, or because the child is inhaling smoke- or fume-filled air, which prevents oxygen entering the lungs.

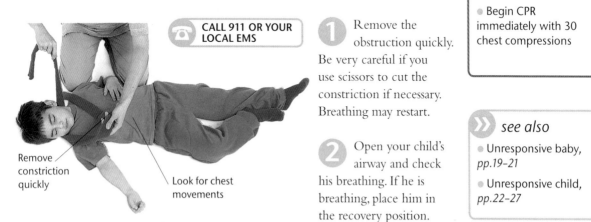

Remove constriction quickly

Look for chest movements

☎ **CALL 911 OR YOUR LOCAL EMS**

1 Remove the obstruction quickly. Be very careful if you use scissors to cut the constriction if necessary. Breathing may restart.

2 Open your child's airway and check his breathing. If he is breathing, place him in the recovery position.

> **! IMPORTANT**
> ● If your child is hanging, support his body while you remove or cut the rope or cord.
> ● Begin CPR immediately with 30 chest compressions

> **» see also**
> ● Unresponsive baby, *pp.19–21*
> ● Unresponsive child, *pp.22–27*

Fume inhalation

Fume, gas, and smoke inhalation requires urgent medical attention as the fumes prevent the child breathing in oxygen. Carbon monoxide prevents tissues taking up oxygen from air breathed in.

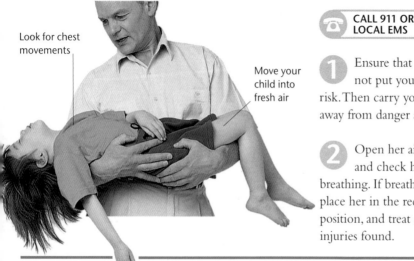

Look for chest movements

Move your child into fresh air

☎ **CALL 911 OR YOUR LOCAL EMS**

1 Ensure that you do not put yourself at risk. Then carry your child away from danger area.

2 Open her airway and check her breathing. If breathing, place her in the recovery position, and treat any injuries found.

> **! IMPORTANT**
> ● **Do not** enter the area if fumes, gas, carbon monoxide, or smoke are still present. CALL FIRE DEPARTMENT and 911.
> ● Begin CPR immediately with 30 chest compressions

> **» see also**
> ● Burns and scalds, *p.52*
> ● Unresponsive baby, *pp.19–21*
> ● Unresponsive child, *pp.22–27*

Croup

This condition is caused by a viral infection. It can be alarming and often occurs at night, but usually passes quickly. Your child will have difficulty breathing, and a short, distinctve barking cough when he breathes out. He may be making a crowing or whistling noise. In a severe attack, he may use muscles around his nose, neck, and upper arms in his attempts to breathe. IF HE HAS blue-tinged skin, CALL 911 OR YOUR LOCAL EMS.

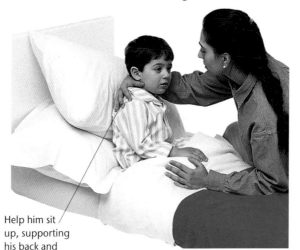

Help him sit up, supporting his back and head

1 Help your child into a comfortable breathing position. Sit him up in bed, propped by pillows, or sit him on your lap supporting his back. Reassure him.

2 Stay calm—if you panic it could frighten the child, which can worsen the attack.

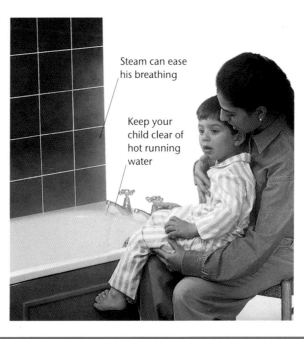

Steam can ease his breathing

Keep your child clear of hot running water

3 If it is safe to do so, create a steamy atmosphere. Take the child into the bathroom, and run a hot faucet or shower, or boil some water in the kitchen.

SEEK MEDICAL ADVICE

Asthma

If your child suffers from asthma, familiarize her with her medication so that she knows how to use it in an attack. You can recognize an attack if your child has difficulty breathing and is coughing; is wheezing, especially when breathing *out;* is distressed and anxious. She may also be tired by efforts to breathe and have a bluish tinge to face and lips.

Sit her in a comfortable position to ease breathing

Lean her forward against a table

If she prefers, sit her on your lap

1 Give your child her usual dose of the medication as soon as an attack starts (see right). Stay calm and reassure her. Tell her to breathe slowly and deeply.

2 Help your child relax. Sit her down in a comfortable position for breathing. This could be leaning forward with her arms resting on a table, or if she prefers, sit her on your lap. Make sure the room is well ventilated and smoke free.

3 If the attack does not ease within a few minutes, give her 1–2 puffs from her medication every two minutes until she has had 6 puffs.

4 If the attack still does not ease,

☎ CALL 911 OR YOUR LOCAL EMS

Using medication

Give your child her medication as soon as an attack starts. Usually if a child has an inhaler she will also have a spacer device to use with it, so use that as well because it's easier to take in the medication. Follow the instructions from your doctor carefully.

Shock

The most likely cause is serious bleeding or a severe burn—injuries that must be treated without delay—dehydration, or a bacterial illness. There could be internal bleeding if shock develops with no visible injury. Early signs are increased respiratory rate and agitation; later signs include pale, cold, and sweaty skin with purplish blotching, bluish lips, rapid pulse becoming weaker, yawning, and thirst; eventually he will be unresponsive.

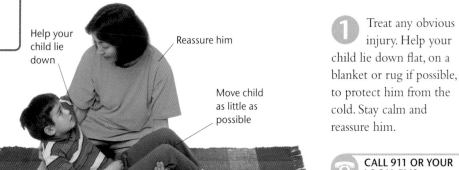

Help your child lie down

Reassure him

Move child as little as possible

1 Treat any obvious injury. Help your child lie down flat, on a blanket or rug if possible, to protect him from the cold. Stay calm and reassure him.

☎ **CALL 911 OR YOUR LOCAL EMS**

2 Keep your child's head low; don't put a pillow under it. Carefully raise your child's legs above the level of his heart to help blood flow to the vital organs; support them on pillows, a chair, or a pile of books padded with a cushion.

Head must be kept low

Raise his legs high above level of his heart

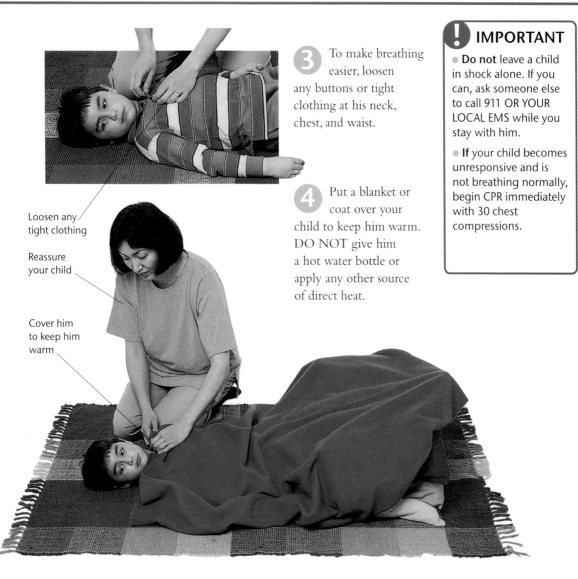

Loosen any tight clothing

Reassure your child

Cover him to keep him warm

3 To make breathing easier, loosen any buttons or tight clothing at his neck, chest, and waist.

4 Put a blanket or coat over your child to keep him warm. DO NOT give him a hot water bottle or apply any other source of direct heat.

> **! IMPORTANT**
>
> ● **Do not** leave a child in shock alone. If you can, ask someone else to call 911 OR YOUR LOCAL EMS while you stay with him.
>
> ● **If** your child becomes unresponsive and is not breathing normally, begin CPR immediately with 30 chest compressions.

Check his pulse rate, and note whether it is strong or weak, regular or irregular

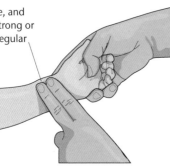

5 Monitor his breathing, pulse, and level of response while you wait for emergency help. Encourage him to talk or answer questions to help you assess any change in his condition. Make a note of any changes and tell the medical personnel.

> **» see also**
>
> ● Severe bleeding, *p.38*
>
> ● Burns and scalds, *p.52*
>
> ● Unresponsive baby, *pp.19–21*
>
> ● Unresponsive child, *pp.22–27*

! IMPORTANT

● **Do not** give anything to eat or drink in case anesthetic is needed.

● **Remove** or cut away clothing to expose a wound if necessary; don't remove anything that is stuck to the wound because it may worsen the bleeding.

● **Do not** apply direct pressure if there is an object embedded in the wound—press on either side of the object to control bleeding.

● **If** the bleeding follows a head injury, and there is thin watery fluid draining from the ears, nose, or an open skull wound, CALL 911 OR YOUR LOCAL EMS.

● **If** your child becomes unresponsive and is not breathing normally, begin CPR with 30 compressions immediately. CALL 911 OR YOUR LOCAL EMS.

≫ see also

● Check circulation, *p.105*

● Dressings, *p.104*

● Embedded object, *p.40*

● Shock, *p.36*

● Unresponsive child, *pp.22–27*

● Triangular bandages, *p.106*

Severe bleeding

Any incident that results in severe bleeding can be very distressing for you and your child. If it is not controlled quickly, a life-threatening condition known as shock will develop. Large wounds may also need stitches.

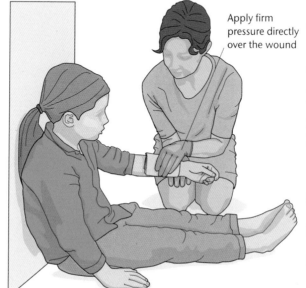

Apply firm pressure directly over the wound

1 Apply direct pressure over the wound immediately, with a clean pad if available, but anything can be used, even a bare hand. Encourage the child to help with this.

2 While you maintain direct pressure, ask a helper to:

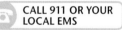
📞 **CALL 911 OR YOUR LOCAL EMS**

Apply a bandage to secure dressing and help maintain direct pressure

3 Secure the dressing with a bandage that is firm enough to maintain pressure, but not so tight that it affects the circulation beyond the bandage. Check the circulation in the hand or foot by pressing the nail. If color does not return right away, the bandage is too tight; if bleeding has stopped, loosen it.

4 Shock is likely to develop if bleeding is severe. Support and elevate the injured part and, while maintaining pressure, help her lie down on a blanket. Raise her legs above the level of her heart. Cover her with another blanket to keep her warm.

When bleeding stops

If the bleeding has stopped and there is no risk of shock, help the child sit down and support an injured hand or arm in an elevation sling for extra comfort on the way to the hospital.

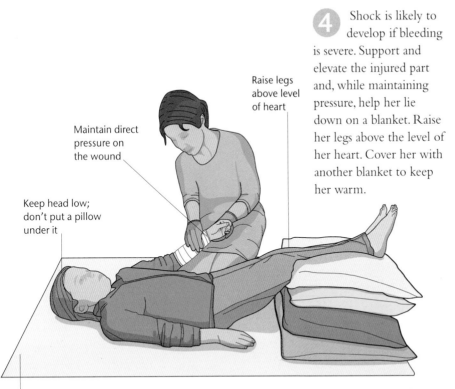

Maintain direct pressure on the wound

Keep head low; don't put a pillow under it

Raise legs above level of heart

Lay child on blanket to protect from cold

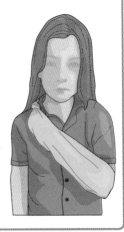

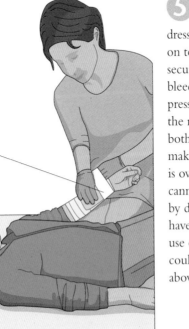

Put a second pad directly over first one and secure with a bandage

5 If bleeding shows through the first dressing, put another pad on top of the first and secure with a bandage. If bleeding continues, direct pressure may not be over the right point. Remove both pads and start again, making sure the new pad is over the wound. If you cannot stop the bleeding by direct pressure and you have been trained in the use of tourniquets, one could be applied 2 inches above the wound.

6 Monitor child's breathing, pulse, and level of response while waiting for emergency help to arrive.

! IMPORTANT

● **Do not** try to remove or dislodge objects that are embedded in a wound because you may cause further damage and bleeding.

Bandaging around larger objects

If the object is very big, build up padding on either side, then bandage above and below the object instead of over the top.

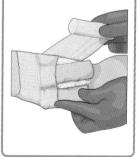

Embedded object

An object such as a piece of glass that becomes stuck in a wound is serious because it may be plugging the wound, preventing bleeding. Do not remove it. Protect it with padding and bandages and get medical help.

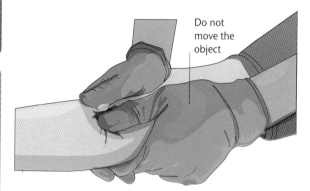

Do not move the object

1 Help your child lie down and keep him calm. If pressure is necessary to slow bleeding, take care not to move the object and cause further damage.

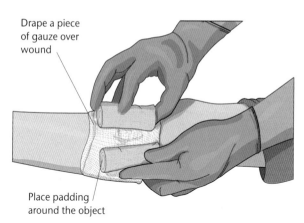

Drape a piece of gauze over wound

Place padding around the object

2 Loosely drape some gauze over the wound and object to minimize the risk of infection. If the object is small, build up padding so that it is slightly higher than the embedded object; spare roller bandages are ideal for this. If the object is large, *see box left*.

Bandage over padding and object

3 Secure padding in place by bandaging over it, being careful not to press down on the embedded object.

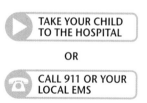

▶ **TAKE YOUR CHILD TO THE HOSPITAL**

OR

☎ **CALL 911 OR YOUR LOCAL EMS**

» *see also*
● Severe bleeding, *p.38*

Cuts and abrasions

Children can be very upset by the tiniest abrasion. Reassure your child and wash the wound. Covering the wound with an adhesive bandage keeps it clean and often makes the child feel better.

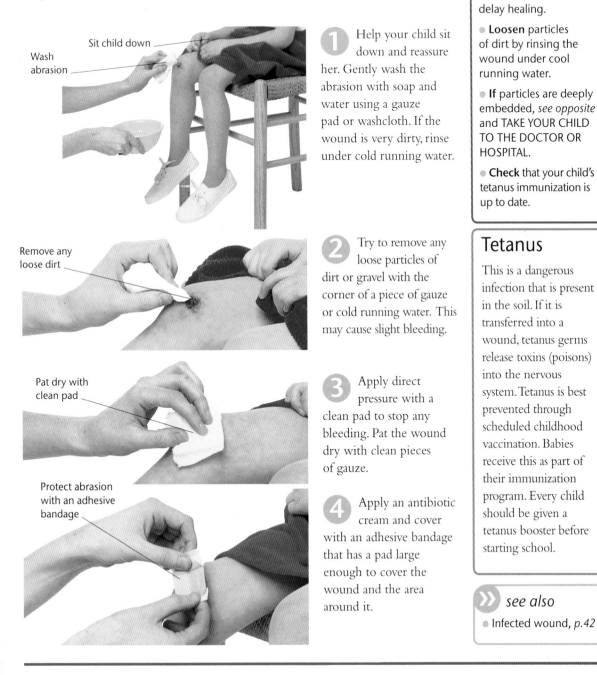

Sit child down

Wash abrasion

1 Help your child sit down and reassure her. Gently wash the abrasion with soap and water using a gauze pad or washcloth. If the wound is very dirty, rinse under cold running water.

Remove any loose dirt

2 Try to remove any loose particles of dirt or gravel with the corner of a piece of gauze or cold running water. This may cause slight bleeding.

Pat dry with clean pad

3 Apply direct pressure with a clean pad to stop any bleeding. Pat the wound dry with clean pieces of gauze.

Protect abrasion with an adhesive bandage

4 Apply an antibiotic cream and cover with an adhesive bandage that has a pad large enough to cover the wound and the area around it.

! IMPORTANT

- **Do not** clean or cover cuts with cotton wool or any fluffy material; it may stick to the wound and delay healing.
- **Loosen** particles of dirt by rinsing the wound under cool running water.
- **If** particles are deeply embedded, *see opposite* and TAKE YOUR CHILD TO THE DOCTOR OR HOSPITAL.
- **Check** that your child's tetanus immunization is up to date.

Tetanus

This is a dangerous infection that is present in the soil. If it is transferred into a wound, tetanus germs release toxins (poisons) into the nervous system. Tetanus is best prevented through scheduled childhood vaccination. Babies receive this as part of their immunization program. Every child should be given a tetanus booster before starting school.

>> *see also*
- Infected wound, *p.42*

Tetanus

This is a dangerous infection caused by a bacterium present in the soil. If these bacteria are transferred into a wound, they may multiply and release toxins (poisons) into the nervous system. Tetanus is best prevented through vaccination. Babies receive this as part of their immunization program. Every child should be given a tetanus booster before starting school.

Infected wound

A wound is infected if there is increasing pain and soreness; swelling, redness, and a feeling of heat around the injury; or there is pus or oozing. If there is an absess or pus draining from the wound, cover it with clean gauze and take your child to the doctor. If there are signs of advanced infection, such as fever, swollen glands, and faint red lines extending from those glands, take your child to the hospital.

1 If red and crusty, apply antibiotic ointment and cover the wound with an adhesive dressing.

2 Cover with clean gauze a wound that has pus or oozing.

TAKE YOUR CHILD TO THE DOCTOR

3 If there are other symptoms of advanced infection,

TAKE YOUR CHILD TO THE HOSPITAL

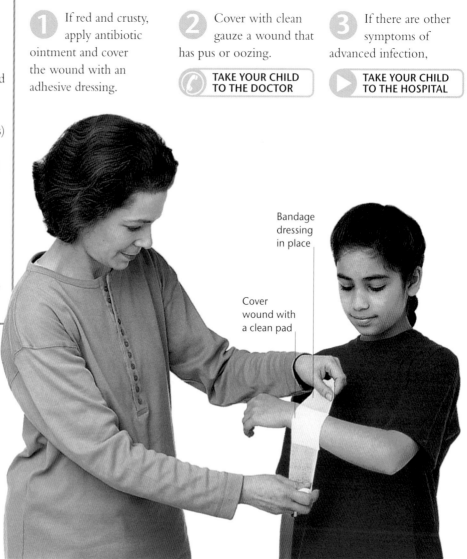

Bandage dressing in place

Cover wound with a clean pad

Blisters

If a blister is caused by friction (for example, a badly fitting shoe), treat as here. You can buy special padded blister bandages.

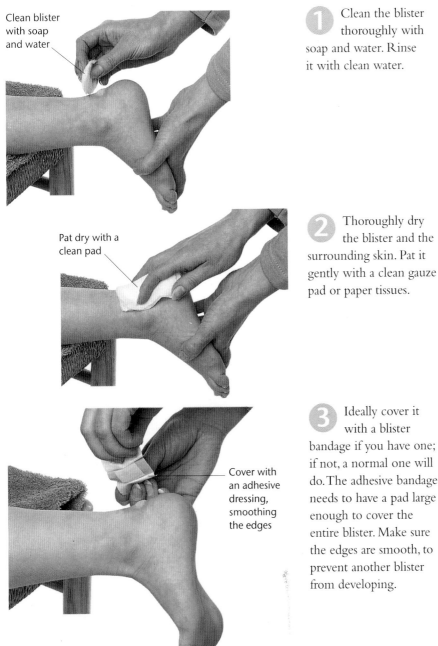

Clean blister with soap and water

1 Clean the blister thoroughly with soap and water. Rinse it with clean water.

Pat dry with a clean pad

2 Thoroughly dry the blister and the surrounding skin. Pat it gently with a clean gauze pad or paper tissues.

Cover with an adhesive dressing, smoothing the edges

3 Ideally cover it with a blister bandage if you have one; if not, a normal one will do. The adhesive bandage needs to have a pad large enough to cover the entire blister. Make sure the edges are smooth, to prevent another blister from developing.

! IMPORTANT

● **If** the blister is very large, cover it with a clean, nonfluffy dressing, held in place with adhesive tape or a bandage.

● **Do not** deliberately break a blister because this can cause it to become infected.

● **Do not** use this method for a blister caused by a burn; treat these as described on pages 52–53.

⟩⟩ *see also*

● Burns and scalds, *p.52*

Eyebrow or eyelid wounds

IMPORTANT

● **Do not** try to remove objects in the eye, except an eyelash or speck of dirt.

● **If** he cannot keep his eyes still, cover both of them.

● **Put** the dressing over the eyebrow and lid, not the eyeball.

A wound to the eyebrow or eyelid may be associated with a more serious eye injury or infection, which can damage the child's sight. If you do not suspect any other injury, follow the steps below, but if there is any chance of eye trauma or objects embedded in the eye, take the child to the hospital immediately.

1 Help your child lie down and cradle his head in your lap to keep it still—make sure he can hear you. He may be in pain; tell him not to rub or move either of his eyes.

2 Reassure your child and lay a sterile dressing over the injured eye. Gently hold the dressing in place until you get medical help.

3 Keep him lying on his back if bleeding.

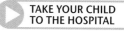
TAKE YOUR CHILD TO THE HOSPITAL

Lay a sterile dressing over injured eye

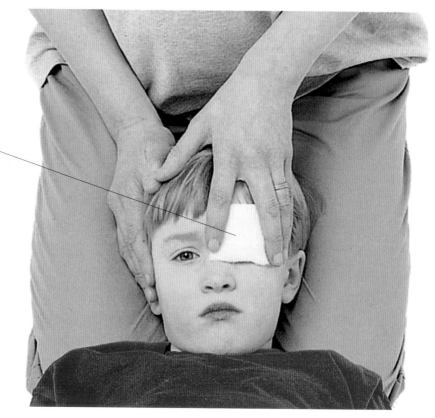

see also

● Chemical burn to eye, *p.56*

● Object in eye, *p.76*

Nosebleed

Children get nosebleeds from a blow to the nose, or from picking it. Bleeding usually stops quickly, but it can alarm young children.

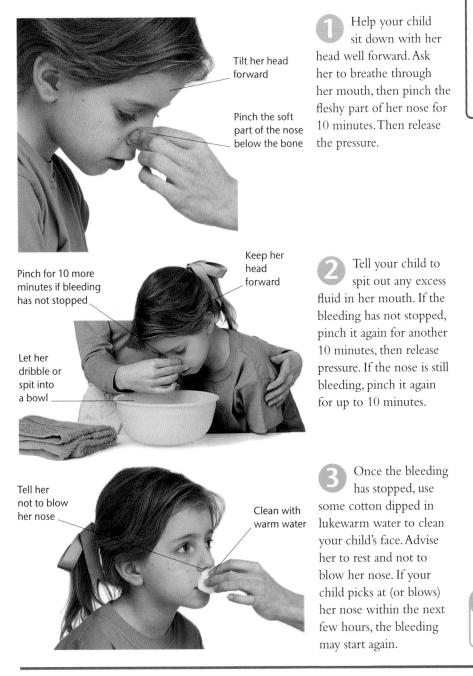

Tilt her head forward

Pinch the soft part of the nose below the bone

1 Help your child sit down with her head well forward. Ask her to breathe through her mouth, then pinch the fleshy part of her nose for 10 minutes. Then release the pressure.

Keep her head forward

Pinch for 10 more minutes if bleeding has not stopped

Let her dribble or spit into a bowl

2 Tell your child to spit out any excess fluid in her mouth. If the bleeding has not stopped, pinch it again for another 10 minutes, then release pressure. If the nose is still bleeding, pinch it again for up to 10 minutes.

Tell her not to blow her nose

Clean with warm water

3 Once the bleeding has stopped, use some cotton dipped in lukewarm water to clean your child's face. Advise her to rest and not to blow her nose. If your child picks at (or blows) her nose within the next few hours, the bleeding may start again.

» *see also*
● Head injury, *p.60*

Ear wound

Outer ear wounds can bleed profusely, which can be alarming. If blood is coming from inside the ear, check that your child has not inserted something into it. If bleeding follows a head injury, CALL 911 OR YOUR LOCAL EMS.

IMPORTANT

● **If** the bleeding follows a head injury and there is blood or watery blood-stained fluid draining from the ear, CALL 911 OR YOUR LOCAL EMS.

● **If** the injury is caused by an earring being ripped out, your child may need stitches. TAKE YOUR CHILD TO THE HOSPITAL.

Bleeding from inside the ear

Help your child into a semiupright position, with his head tilted toward the injured side to allow blood to drain away. Put an absorbent pad over the ear and bandage it lightly in place. Do not plug the ear. SEEK MEDICAL ADVICE.

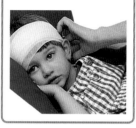

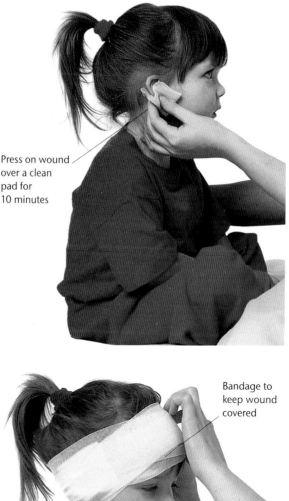

Press on wound over a clean pad for 10 minutes

1 Help your child sit down and gently pinch the wound with your thumb and forefinger over a clean piece of gauze. Keep pressing for 10 minutes.

Bandage to keep wound covered

2 Cover the injured ear with a sterile dressing and lightly bandage it in place.

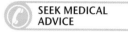
SEEK MEDICAL ADVICE

» see also
● Head injury, p.60
● Object in ear, p.77

Mouth wound

These wounds can be the result of a child biting the inside of his mouth in a fall, for example, or from the loss of a tooth. Make sure your child does not inhale blood because this can result in breathing problems.

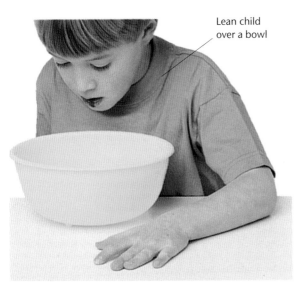

Lean child over a bowl

1 Help your child sit down with his head over a bowl. Encourage him to spit out any blood.

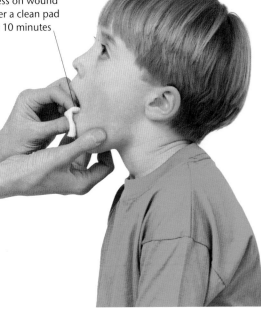

Press on wound over a clean pad for 10 minutes

2 Place a pad over the wound and pinch it between your thumb and forefinger, maintaining the pressure for 10 minutes. Your child may be able to do this for himself.

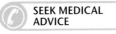

SEEK MEDICAL ADVICE

! IMPORTANT

● Do not wash out his mouth—it may disturb a blood clot.

● If he loses an "adult" tooth, it may be possible for a dentist to replant it. Do not clean the tooth. Keep it moist by putting the tooth in milk or saliva. Take your child to the dentist.

● Ensure a baby tooth has not been inhaled or swallowed. A dentist should check the gum.

Bleeding from tooth socket

Ask your child to sit down and support her jaw. Place a pad over the tooth socket, making sure that it is higher than the adjacent teeth. Tell her to bite hard on the pad. A younger child may need you to hold the pad in place.

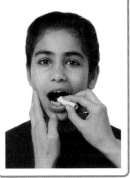

Care of the amputated part

Preserve the severed part until you get to the hospital. Wrap it in plastic wrap or a plastic bag, then in a soft fabric, such as a cotton handkerchief or piece of gauze. Place the wrapped part in a plastic bag filled with ice cubes; the part must not touch the ice. Put the whole package in another bag or container. Mark with the time of injury and the child's name then give it to the emergency personnel.

Amputation

Whether a injury causes partial or total amputation, the limb can often be reattached. Your child will need an anaesthetic so don't give him anything to eat or drink because it may delay surgery.

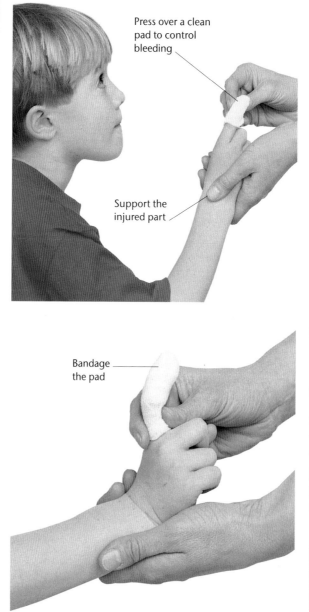

Press over a clean pad to control bleeding

Support the injured part

Bandage the pad

1 Control the blood loss by pressing firmly on the injury using a sterile dressing or clean pad. If necessary, treat for shock; help your child lie down and raise his legs above his heart.

2 Bandage or tape the dressing firmly in place. You can cover a finger with a gauze finger bandage to protect it.

📞 **CALL 911 OR YOUR LOCAL EMS**

3 Tell the 911 operator or EMS dispatcher it is an amputation. Monitor your child for signs of shock while waiting. If possible, put the severed part in a plastic bag and keep it cool, *see left*.

» see also
● Severe bleeding, *p.38*
● Shock, *p.36*

Internal bleeding

Suspect this when signs of shock develop without obvious blood loss. There may also be "pattern bruising" around the injury with marks from clothes or crushing objects because bleeding may be occurring in the lungs or abdomen.

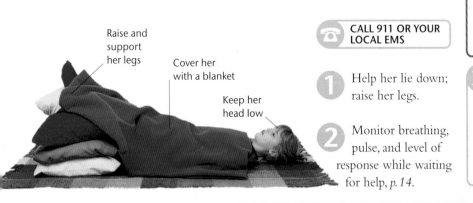

Raise and support her legs

Cover her with a blanket

Keep her head low

> **!** **IMPORTANT**
> ● **If** the child is unresponsive, open her airway and check breathing. If breathing, place in the recovery position; if she is not breathing, begin CPR immediately with 30 chest compressions.

☎ **CALL 911 OR YOUR LOCAL EMS**

1 Help her lie down; raise her legs.

2 Monitor breathing, pulse, and level of response while waiting for help, *p.14*.

>> *see also*
● Shock, *p.36*
● Unresponsive baby, *pp.19–21*
● Unresponsive child, *pp.22–27*

Crush injury

A crush injury can be serious because it may cause internal bleeding and broken bones as well as open wounds.

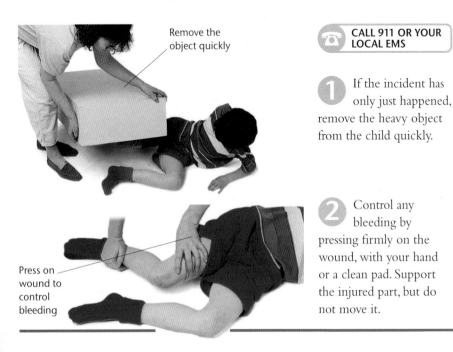

Remove the object quickly

Press on wound to control bleeding

☎ **CALL 911 OR YOUR LOCAL EMS**

1 If the incident has only just happened, remove the heavy object from the child quickly.

2 Control any bleeding by pressing firmly on the wound, with your hand or a clean pad. Support the injured part, but do not move it.

> **!** **IMPORTANT**
> ● **If** your child has been crushed for over 30 minutes, do not remove the object—it may cause toxic fluids from the damaged muscles to be released into the body. This increases the risk of death.
>
> ● **If** you suspect broken bones, support the injury, but do not move your child unless he is in immediate danger and it is safe to do so. Watch for signs of shock while waiting for help.

>> *see also*
● Severe bleeding, *p.38*
● Shock, *p.36*
● Leg injury, *p.64*

ⓘ IMPORTANT

● **Monitor** your child for signs of shock.

● **If** your child becomes unresponsive and is not breathing normally, begin CPR with 30 compressions immediately. CALL 911 OR YOUR LOCAL EMS.

● **If** you need to place him in the recovery position, place him so that he is lying on his injured side to support his chest and help the good lung function.

Chest wound

A wound to the chest can cause serious internal injuries. The lungs are particularly vulnerable, and breathing problems, shock, and collapsed lungs may follow an injury. If the wound is not obviously bleeding, leave it exposed—don't cover it with a dresssing.

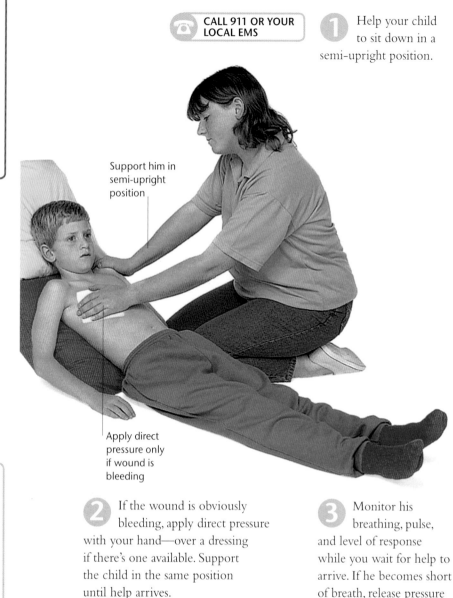

☎ **CALL 911 OR YOUR LOCAL EMS**

1 Help your child to sit down in a semi-upright position.

Support him in semi-upright position

Apply direct pressure only if wound is bleeding

2 If the wound is obviously bleeding, apply direct pressure with your hand—over a dressing if there's one available. Support the child in the same position until help arrives.

3 Monitor his breathing, pulse, and level of response while you wait for help to arrive. If he becomes short of breath, release pressure and remove dressing.

⟫ see also

● Checking vital signs, *p.14*

● Severe bleeding, *p.38*

● Shock, *p.36*

● Unresponsive child, *pp.22–27*

Abdominal wound

A child with an abdominal wound is likely to develop the signs of shock. There is high risk of internal as well as external bleeding because internal organs may be damaged, so this is an emergency.

! IMPORTANT

● **Monitor** your child for signs of shock.

● **If** your child becomes unresponsive and is not breathing normally, begin CPR with 30 compressions immediately. CALL 911 OR YOUR LOCAL EMS.

● **If** intestines are protruding from wound, do not apply pressure. Follow steps 2–4.

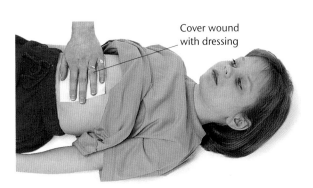

Cover wound with dressing

1 Help your child lie down and loosen any tight clothing around her waist. Cover the injury with a large sterile dressing and, if needed to stop bleeding, apply pressure over the pad.

☎ **CALL 911 OR YOUR LOCAL EMS**

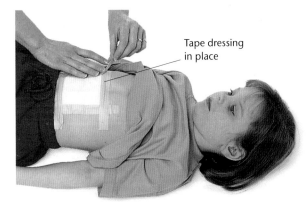

Tape dressing in place

2 If your child has a major abdominal wound, just cover the wound with a sterile dressing. Raise and support her knees by placing a pillow under them—this eases the strain on the abdomen.

3 Secure the dressing lightly in place with tape; use hypoallergenic tape if possible.

4 Monitor her breathing, pulse, and level of response while you wait for help to arrive. Treat for shock if necessary. Continue to reassure her and watch for any change in her condition while waiting for help.

»» see also

● Checking vital signs, *p.14*

● Severe bleeding, *p.38*

● Shock, *p.36*

● Unresponsive child, *pp.22–27*

Burns and scalds

It is very important to cool the burn as quickly as possible to stop the burning, minimize damage, and reduce pain. You must always seek medical advice or take a child to the hospital following any burn—however small—because there is high risk of infection.

Thermal burns to the mouth and throat

Burns in this area are very serious as they cause swelling and inflammation of the air passages, giving a serious risk of suffocation. Act quickly. If necessary, loosen clothing from around her neck.

• **If** your child becomes unresponsive and is not breathing normally, begin CPR with 30 compressions immediately. CALL 911 OR YOUR LOCAL EMS.

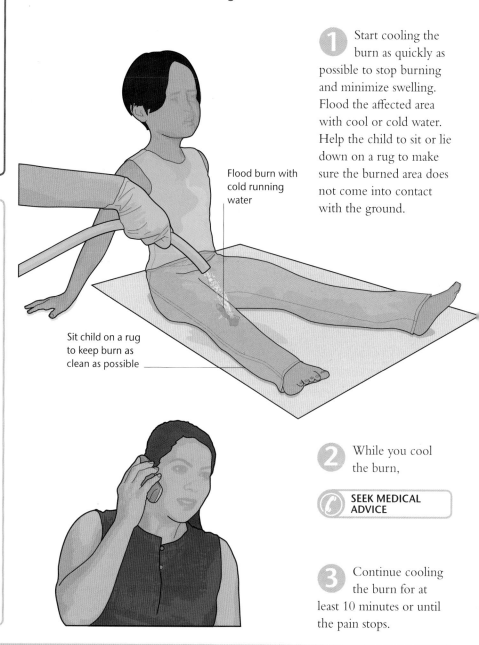

Flood burn with cold running water

Sit child on a rug to keep burn as clean as possible

1 Start cooling the burn as quickly as possible to stop burning and minimize swelling. Flood the affected area with cool or cold water. Help the child to sit or lie down on a rug to make sure the burned area does not come into contact with the ground.

2 While you cool the burn,

SEEK MEDICAL ADVICE

3 Continue cooling the burn for at least 10 minutes or until the pain stops.

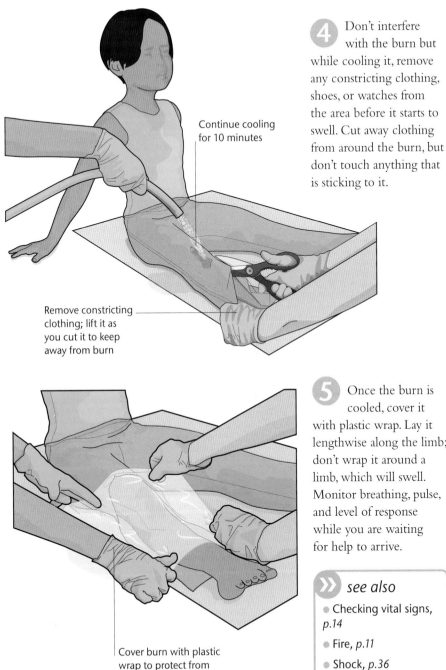

Continue cooling for 10 minutes

Remove constricting clothing; lift it as you cut it to keep away from burn

Cover burn with plastic wrap to protect from infection

④ Don't interfere with the burn but while cooling it, remove any constricting clothing, shoes, or watches from the area before it starts to swell. Cut away clothing from around the burn, but don't touch anything that is sticking to it.

⑤ Once the burn is cooled, cover it with plastic wrap. Lay it lengthwise along the limb; don't wrap it around a limb, which will swell. Monitor breathing, pulse, and level of response while you are waiting for help to arrive.

》》 see also
- Checking vital signs, *p.14*
- Fire, *p.11*
- Shock, *p.36*
- Unresponsive baby, *pp.19–21*
- Unresponsive child, *pp.22–27*

❗ IMPORTANT

- **Do not** remove any clothing or material that is sticking to the burned area because this may cause further injury.

- **If** you have no plastic wrap, use a sterile dressing or any clean, nonfluffy material.

- **Do not** give your child anything to eat or drink because an anesthetic may be needed.

- **If** your child becomes unresponsive and is not breathing normally, begin CPR with 30 compressions immediately. CALL 911 OR YOUR LOCAL EMS.

Using a plastic bag

You can use a clean plastic bag to protect an injured hand or foot. Secure it loosely with a piece of tape that is applied to the bag; don't put tape on the child's skin.

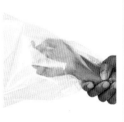

! IMPORTANT

● **Do not** touch your child until you are sure the electrical current has been turned off.

● **Seek** medical advice for all burns to children.

● **Do not** use cold water; a small child could become hypothermic.

● **If** child becomes unresponsive and is not breathing normally, begin CPR immediately with 30 chest compressions; if breathing, place in the recovery position. CALL 911 OR YOUR LOCAL EMS.

Electrical burn

An electric shock from a low-voltage source can result in burns. These may occur at both the point of entry and the point of exit of the current.

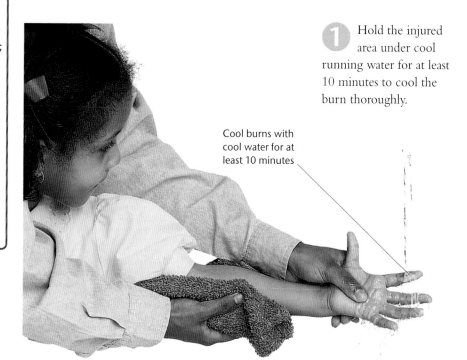

1 Hold the injured area under cool running water for at least 10 minutes to cool the burn thoroughly.

Cool burns with cool water for at least 10 minutes

Cover burns on a hand with a clean plastic bag

2 If the burn is on a hand or foot, a clean plastic bag can be used, bandaged below the burn, or clean material such as a pillowcase.

▶ **TAKE YOUR CHILD TO THE HOSPITAL**

» see also

● Electrical injury, *p.12*

● Unresponsive baby, *pp.19–21*

● Unresponsive child, *p.22–27*

Chemical burn to skin

Chemical burns can be caused by household agents such as oven cleaner or paint stripper. These burns can be serious and there will be fierce, stinging pain, redness or staining, followed by blistering and peeling of skin.

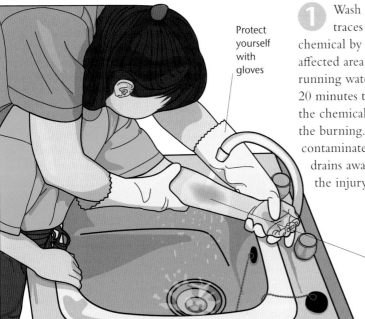

Protect yourself with gloves

1 Wash away all traces of the chemical by holding the affected area under cool running water for at least 20 minutes to remove the chemicals and stop the burning. Make sure contaminated water drains away from the injury.

Wash chemical off under cold running water for at least 20 minutes

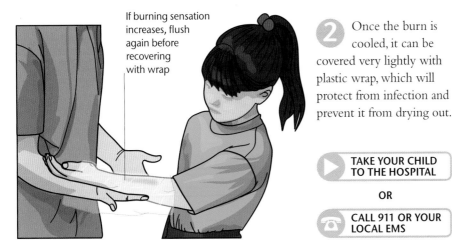

If burning sensation increases, flush again before recovering with wrap

2 Once the burn is cooled, it can be covered very lightly with plastic wrap, which will protect from infection and prevent it from drying out.

▶ **TAKE YOUR CHILD TO THE HOSPITAL**

OR

☎ **CALL 911 OR YOUR LOCAL EMS**

! IMPORTANT

● **Call** Poison Control Center (800-222-1222) for guidance.

● **Note** the name of the substance that caused the burn and give the information to the hospital staff.

● **Always** wear protective gloves when treating your child, and beware of chemical fumes.

● **If** plastic wrap is not available, a clean, nonfluffy material can be laid over the burn to protect from infection.

≫ see also

● Chemical burn to eye, *p.56*

● Fume inhalation, *p.33*

● Swallowed chemicals, *p.57*

! IMPORTANT

- **Do not** let your child touch his eye. The eye will be shut in spasm and pain, so gently pull the eyelids open.

Chemical burn to eye

Splashes of chemicals in the eye can cause scarring or even blindness. Your child may have a chemical burn if he complains of fierce pain in the eye; he has difficulty opening the affected eye; the surface of the eye is watery; or there is redness and swelling in and around the eye.

Using pitcher of water

If you can't hold your child under a faucet, you may find it easier to use a pitcher to pour water over the affected eye. Get a helper to support your child with her head tilted down and to one side. Do not splash the unaffected eye with the contaminated water.

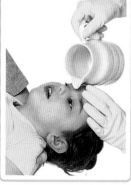

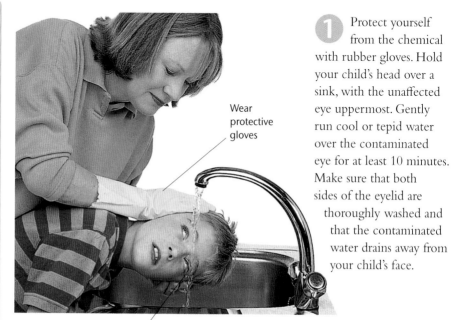

Wear protective gloves

Rinse eye with cold water for 10 minutes

1 Protect yourself from the chemical with rubber gloves. Hold your child's head over a sink, with the unaffected eye uppermost. Gently run cool or tepid water over the contaminated eye for at least 10 minutes. Make sure that both sides of the eyelid are thoroughly washed and that the contaminated water drains away from your child's face.

Cover eye with clean pad

2 Once the injured eye is thoroughly washed, cover it with a large sterile dressing. Hold the dressing in place until you get medical aid.

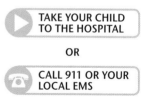

▶ **TAKE YOUR CHILD TO THE HOSPITAL**

OR

☎ **CALL 911 OR YOUR LOCAL EMS**

Swallowed chemicals

If you think your child has swallowed a poison, try to find out what, when, and how much she has taken. Be aware too that some chemicals also give off dangerous fumes.

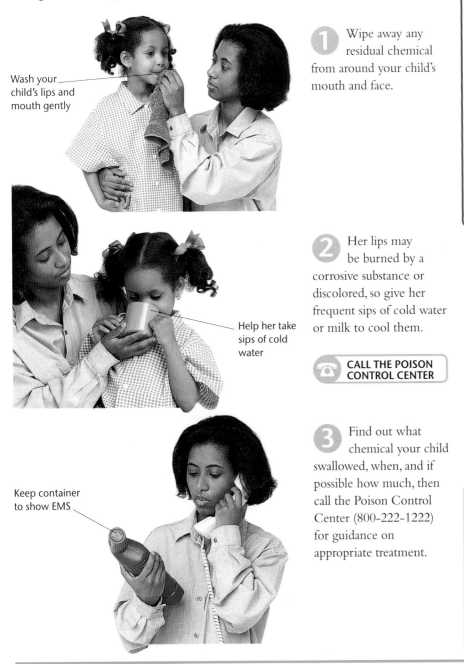

Wash your child's lips and mouth gently

1 Wipe away any residual chemical from around your child's mouth and face.

Help her take sips of cold water

2 Her lips may be burned by a corrosive substance or discolored, so give her frequent sips of cold water or milk to cool them.

☎ **CALL THE POISON CONTROL CENTER**

Keep container to show EMS

3 Find out what chemical your child swallowed, when, and if possible how much, then call the Poison Control Center (800-222-1222) for guidance on appropriate treatment.

> **!** **IMPORTANT**
>
> ● **Do not** try to make your child vomit because this can cause further harm.
>
> ● **If** your child becomes unresponsive, open her airway and check for breathing. If breathing, put her in the recovery position. If not breathing, begin CPR immediately. CALL 911.
>
> ● **If** you need to give rescue breaths and there are chemicals on the child's mouth, protect yourself by using a face shield or pocket mask.

>> *see also*
- Chemical burn to eye, *opposite*
- Fume inhalation, *p.33*
- Unresponsive baby, *pp.19–21*
- Unresponsive child, *pp.22–27*

Drug or alcohol poisoning

» see also

● Unresponsive baby, pp.19–21

● Unresponsive child, pp.22–27

If your child has taken medication, the container may be nearby. If he drank alcohol, there may be a smell of alcohol and he may be staggering and throw up. He may also have a flushed and moist face; slurred speech; deep, noisy breathing; and a pounding pulse.

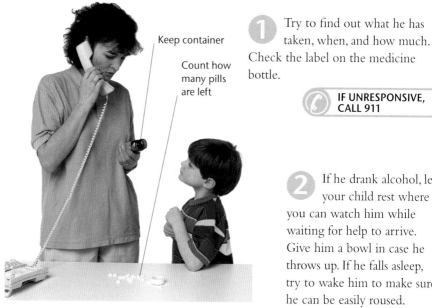

Keep container

Count how many pills are left

1 Try to find out what he has taken, when, and how much. Check the label on the medicine bottle.

IF UNRESPONSIVE, CALL 911

2 If he drank alcohol, let your child rest where you can watch him while waiting for help to arrive. Give him a bowl in case he throws up. If he falls asleep, try to wake him to make sure he can be easily roused.

Plant poisoning

Many plants are poisonous in large quantities. Small pieces or one or two berries are unlikely to be fatal but can cause stomach upset.

Check his mouth and tell him to spit out any pieces

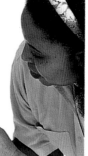

1 Try to find out what your child ate, when, and how much—keep a sample of the plant.

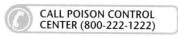
CALL POISON CONTROL CENTER (800-222-1222)

2 Look inside your child's mouth. Pick out any remaining pieces of plant or berries.

Scalp wound

This type of wound can bleed profusely. If the wound was caused by a blow to the child's head, watch for any change in her condition, especially her level of response, while waiting for emergency help.

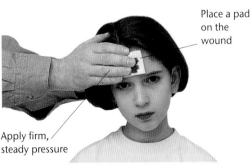

Place a pad on the wound

Apply firm, steady pressure

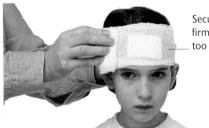

Secure bandage firmly but not too tightly

Keep her head and shoulders slightly raised

1 Cover the injury with a clean pad or sterile dressing that is larger than the wound. Press firmly on the pad and the wound to control the bleeding. Place another pad on top, if necessary, and keep pressing on the wound.

2 Bandage the dressing firmly in place. If the bleeding continues, apply pressure again with your hand.

3 Help your child lie down with her head and shoulders slightly raised.

4 If you think the wound may need stitches, take your child to the doctor or emergency room.

> **! IMPORTANT**
>
> ● **If** blood continues to seep through the first and second dressings, add another and apply more pressure to stop the bleeding.
>
> ● **If** the bleeding is massive, uncontrollable, or there is a chance of brain injury, **call 911 or your local EMS.**
>
> ● **If** your child becomes unresponsive and is not breathing normally, begin CPR immediately with 30 chest compressions. CALL 911 OR YOUR LOCAL EMS.

> **»** *see also*
>
> ● Head injury, *p.60*
> ● Severe bleeding, *p.38*
> ● Shock, *p.36*
> ● Unresponsive baby, *pp.19–21*
> ● Unresponsive child, *pp.22–27*

! **IMPORTANT**

! **IMPORTANT**

● **Never** shake a baby or child to assess her reactions.

● **If** a head injury occurs during an athletic activity, do not allow your child to continue to play until she has been assessed by a healthcare professional.

Signs of worsening head injury

Seek urgent medical advice if after a head injury you notice any of the following in your child:

● She becomes disoriented and/or increasingly drowsy;

● She complains of double vision;

● She is vomiting;

● She complains of a persistent headache;

● She is confused, with loss of memory, dizziness;

● She has difficulty speaking and/or walking and problems with balance;

● She suffers a seizure.

Head injury

If your child has a minor bump to the head, she may simply have a bruise with no other sign of injury. If, however, the child has suffered a more serious blow, the brain can be shaken inside the skull and she may be dazed or temporarily unresponsive—this is concussion. Your child may have a headache, feel dizzy, complain of nausea, and may not remember what happened.

If there has been a severe blow to the head, there may be bleeding or swelling within the skull that can press on the brain, which is a serious condition. A child may seem unaffected at first, but as time goes by (minutes, hours, or even days) her condition can worsen, and so it is very important to watch her and monitor her condition looking for signs of a worsening head injury (*see box, left*).

1 If the child is dazed, help her lie down on the floor (protect her from the cold). Don't sit her on a chair because she may fall off and hurt herself.

2 If your child was "knocked out," even briefly,

SEEK MEDICAL ADVICE

3 Make her rest and watch her closely. Check her for signs of a worsening head injury, *left*, reassure her, and stay with her. If she does not recover completely or shows any sign of deterioration,

☎ **CALL 911 OR YOUR LOCAL EMS**

Remain with her and monitor her condition

Help her to sit on the floor, not on a chair

Checking a child's level of response

Your child could be awake following an injury, completely unresponsive, or somewhere between the two. She may deteriorate over minutes, hours, or even days. It is important to assess her condition and monitor any changes so that you can tell the emergency personnel or hospital staff.

● Is she alert? Are her eyes open and does she respond normally when you talk to her?

● Does she only respond to voice by answering simple questions or obeying instructions? Does she open her eyes?

● Does she respond only to pain, for example, by opening her eyes if you flick her foot or tap her shoulder?

● Is she completely unresponsive?

Note any response or change of response, and the time.

> **! IMPORTANT**

● **Suspect** skull fracture if the level of response is impaired, there is blood or blood-stained watery fluid coming from the nose or ear; there is a soft area on the scalp; blood showing on the white of the eye; and/or distortion of the face or head.

● **Remember,** there's a possibility of a spinal injury with any head injury.

If your child becomes unresponsive

Do not move your child because there could be an associated back or neck injury, and moving her could result in damage to the brain or spinal cord.

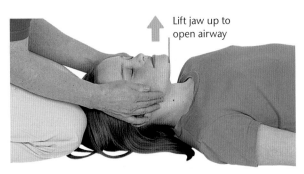

Lift jaw up to open airway

1 Kneel behind her head and rest your elbows on the ground or your knees. Open her airway using the jaw thrust: place one hand on either side of her face, with your fingertips on the angles of her jaw. Gently lift the jaw up to open the airway (don't tilt her head back).

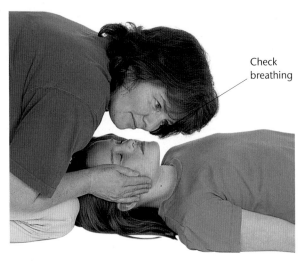

Check breathing

2 Check her breathing. If she is breathing, continue to support her jaw to keep the airway open. If she is not breathing, begin CPR immediately. Ask someone else to call 911.

☎ **CALL 911 OR YOUR LOCAL EMS**

>> *see also*

● Checking vital signs, *p.14*

● Cold packs, *p.108*

● Scalp wound, *p.59*

● Spine injury, *p.63*

● Unresponsive baby, *pp.19–21*

● Unresponsive child, *pp.22–27*

! **IMPORTANT**

● **If** pinching her nose hurts too much, simply ask her to sit forward over the bowl and give her a soft pad or towel to soak up the blood.

» *see also*

● Nosebleed, *p.45*

● Unresponsive baby, *pp.19–21*

● Unresponsive child, *pp.22–27*

Nose or cheekbone injury

The main risk with fractures to the nose or cheekbones is that the swelling can affect the air passages, causing breathing problems. There may also be bleeding from the child's nose or mouth.

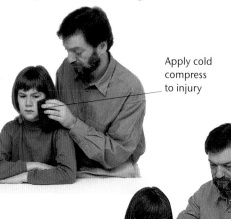

Apply cold compress to injury

Pinch nostrils together to stop bleeding

1 Help your child sit down and apply a cold pack (see *p.108*) to the injured area to help minimize the swelling. Hold the cold pack in place for about 20 minutes.

2 If your child's nose is bleeding, ask her to sit with her head well forward and to pinch the fleshy part of her nose to help control bleeding. If any bones are broken,

▶ **TAKE YOUR CHILD TO THE HOSPITAL**

! **IMPORTANT**

● **If** your child becomes unresponsive and is not breathing normally, begin CPR immediately with 30 chest compressions. CALL 911 OR YOUR LOCAL EMS.

» *see also*

● Unresponsive baby, *pp.19–21*

● Unresponsive child, *p.22–27*

Jaw injury

A broken jaw will be tender and swollen, with loss of normal mobility. Her teeth may be out of line.

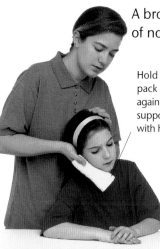

Hold ice pack in cloth against jaw; support jaw with hand

1 Help your child to sit with head well forward. Tell her to spit out any loose teeth and not to swallow any blood or saliva.

2 Hold an icepack gently under her injured jaw, and support it in this position until you get to the hospital. Do not bandage the pad in place in case she vomits.

▶ **TAKE YOUR CHILD TO THE HOSPITAL**

Spine injury

If a child lands on his neck or back in a fall or falls awkwardly and complains of back pain or tingling in any part of his body, suspect spine injury. Support him in the position found to prevent further damage.

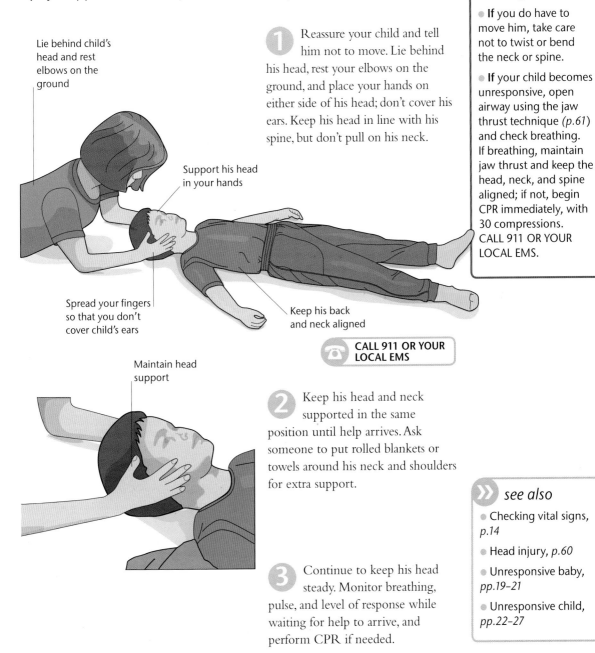

Lie behind child's head and rest elbows on the ground

Support his head in your hands

Spread your fingers so that you don't cover child's ears

Keep his back and neck aligned

Maintain head support

1 Reassure your child and tell him not to move. Lie behind his head, rest your elbows on the ground, and place your hands on either side of his head; don't cover his ears. Keep his head in line with his spine, but don't pull on his neck.

☎ **CALL 911 OR YOUR LOCAL EMS**

2 Keep his head and neck supported in the same position until help arrives. Ask someone to put rolled blankets or towels around his neck and shoulders for extra support.

3 Continue to keep his head steady. Monitor breathing, pulse, and level of response while waiting for help to arrive, and perform CPR if needed.

❗ IMPORTANT

● **Do not** move the injured child from the position in which you find him unless his life is in danger.

● **If** you do have to move him, take care not to twist or bend the neck or spine.

● **If** your child becomes unresponsive, open airway using the jaw thrust technique *(p.61)* and check breathing. If breathing, maintain jaw thrust and keep the head, neck, and spine aligned; if not, begin CPR immediately, with 30 compressions. CALL 911 OR YOUR LOCAL EMS.

» *see also*

● Checking vital signs, *p.14*

● Head injury, *p.60*

● Unresponsive baby, *pp.19–21*

● Unresponsive child, *pp.22–27*

Pelvic injury

If your child has a broken pelvis, she will be unable to stand, with pain around the hip and groin, and possible bleeding from the urinary orifice.

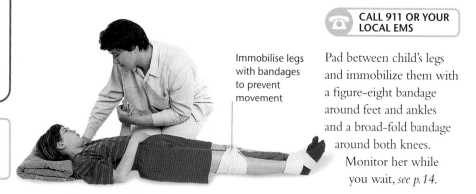

Immobilise legs with bandages to prevent movement

Pad between child's legs and immobilize them with a figure-eight bandage around feet and ankles and a broad-fold bandage around both knees. Monitor her while you wait, *see p.14.*

IMPORTANT

● **Do not** move your child—treat her in the position you found her.

● **Do not** bandage if it causes pain.

● **If** you see signs of shock or bleeding but no obvious wound, treat for shock but do not raise her legs.

>> *see also*
● Shock, *p.36*

Leg injury

Suspect a break if your child is in severe pain. He needs an X-ray or scan to confirm whether or not a bone is broken. Treat the leg in the position found to prevent broken bone ends causing further internal injury.

IMPORTANT

● **If** there is a wound, treat bleeding and cover with a sterile dressing.

● **Do not** attempt to straighten the injured leg.

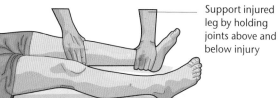

Support injured leg by holding joints above and below injury

1 Make your child comfortable and keep him still. Keep his leg in the position you found it by supporting the ankle and knee joints.

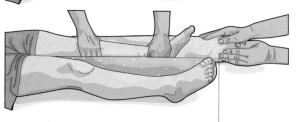

Place rolled blankets or towels around injured leg

2 Support the joints until help arrives. Ask a helper to place padding along the outer side of the limb and between the legs. Cover your child with another blanket to keep him warm. If you suspect shock, raise only the *uninjured* leg.

>> *see also*
● Severe bleeding, *p.38*
● Shock, *p.36*

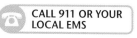

How to splint an injured leg

If you are going to have to wait for help, for example if you are in a remote area, you can splint the injured leg for extra support.

1 Maintain support at the joints. Ask a helper to place padding such as a rolled-up towel or small blanket between the thighs, knees, and ankles. Bring the *uninjured* leg to the broken one.

2 Slide bandages through the hollows under the legs. Place a narrow-fold bandage at the ankle and broad-fold bandages under the knees and below the fracture. Secure the bandage at the ankles first.

3 Secure the broad-fold bandages at the knee then below the injury site—and above if there is room. Tie all knots against the *uninjured* leg.

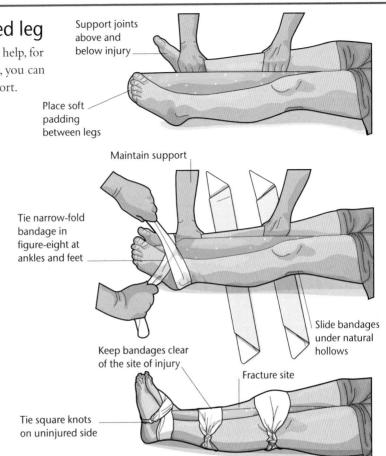

Support joints above and below injury

Place soft padding between legs

Maintain support

Tie narrow-fold bandage in figure-eight at ankles and feet

Slide bandages under natural hollows

Keep bandages clear of the site of injury

Fracture site

Tie square knots on uninjured side

Making broad-fold and narrow-fold bandages

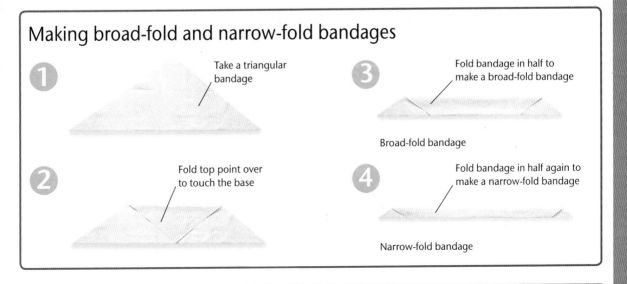

1 Take a triangular bandage

2 Fold top point over to touch the base

3 Fold bandage in half to make a broad-fold bandage

Broad-fold bandage

4 Fold bandage in half again to make a narrow-fold bandage

Narrow-fold bandage

Knee injury

This type of injury can be very painful, and your child may not be able to move it. The area around the knee joint can swell very quickly.

»» see also

● Cold packs, *p.108*

● Leg injury, *p.64*

Support his knee with a pillow

Wrap padding around joint

Secure padding with bandage

Keep him comfortable

1 Reassure your child and help him lie down. Place a pillow under his legs to support them in the most comfortable position. Place a cold pack on the knee. Then wrap a layer of soft padding around it.

2 Secure the padding with a bandage.

SEEK MEDICAL ADVICE

Foot injury

Your child's foot may be bruised, swollen, and stiff and she may not be able to stand. If caused by crushing, one or more bones may be broken.

»» see also

● Cold packs, *p.108*

● Leg injury, *p.64*

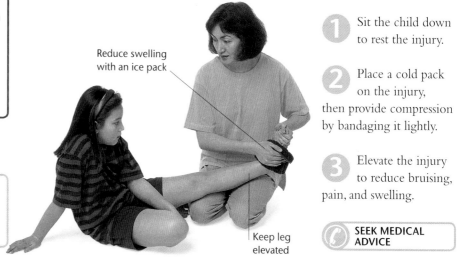

Reduce swelling with an ice pack

Keep leg elevated

1 Sit the child down to rest the injury.

2 Place a cold pack on the injury, then provide compression by bandaging it lightly.

3 Elevate the injury to reduce bruising, pain, and swelling.

SEEK MEDICAL ADVICE

Ankle injury

The most common injury is a sprain. Suspect a sprain if your child can't take her full weight on her foot after a fall, or she has twisted, or wrenched, her ankle. She may need an X-ray or scan.

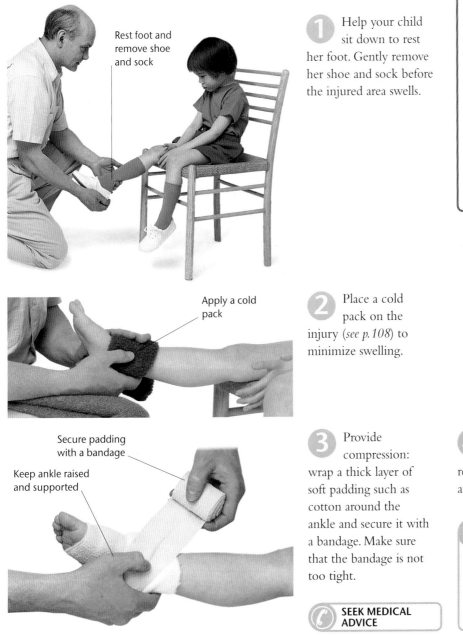

Rest foot and remove shoe and sock

Apply a cold pack

Secure padding with a bandage

Keep ankle raised and supported

1 Help your child sit down to rest her foot. Gently remove her shoe and sock before the injured area swells.

2 Place a cold pack on the injury (*see p. 108*) to minimize swelling.

3 Provide compression: wrap a thick layer of soft padding such as cotton around the ankle and secure it with a bandage. Make sure that the bandage is not too tight.

SEEK MEDICAL ADVICE

4 Elevate the injury to help reduce bruising, pain, and swelling.

> **see also**
> ● Check circulation, *p.105*
> ● Cold packs, *p.108*
> ● Leg injury, *p.64*

! IMPORTANT

● **If** the pain is very severe or you think a bone could be broken, wrap the ankle as shown below and TAKE YOUR CHILD TO THE HOSPITAL or CALL 911.

● Follow the RICE procedure:

R Rest injured part.

I Place ice on the injury.

C Apply **compression** by loosely bandaging the injured part.

E Elevate injured part.

! **IMPORTANT**

● **If** putting a sling on the child causes further pain, stop and support the affected arm by hand instead.

Collarbone injury

A collarbone may be broken by indirect force, for example, if a child falls onto her outstretched hand, or by a blow to her shoulder. There will be tenderness in your child's shoulder and arm—increased by attempts to move it—and her head may be turned and inclined to the injured side.

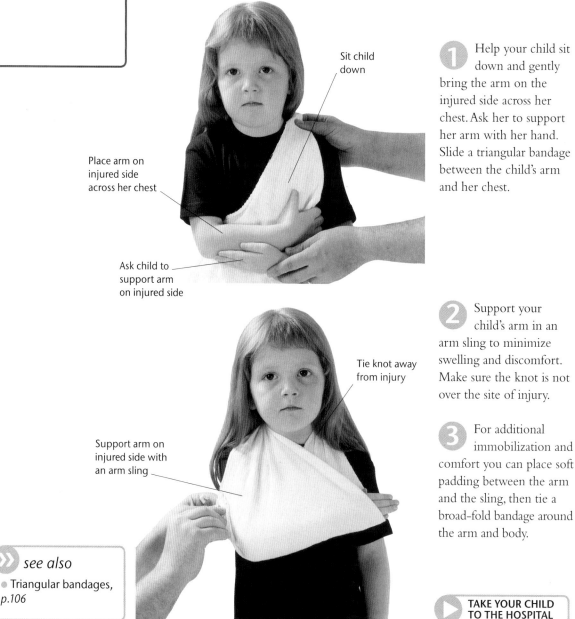

Sit child down

Place arm on injured side across her chest

Ask child to support arm on injured side

Tie knot away from injury

Support arm on injured side with an arm sling

1 Help your child sit down and gently bring the arm on the injured side across her chest. Ask her to support her arm with her hand. Slide a triangular bandage between the child's arm and her chest.

2 Support your child's arm in an arm sling to minimize swelling and discomfort. Make sure the knot is not over the site of injury.

3 For additional immobilization and comfort you can place soft padding between the arm and the sling, then tie a broad-fold bandage around the arm and body.

» *see also*
● Triangular bandages, *p.106*

▶ **TAKE YOUR CHILD TO THE HOSPITAL**

Rib injury

A child may have a broken rib following a blow to her chest, a heavy fall, or having been crushed. Symptoms include sharp pain at the fracture site, bruising, swelling, or possible wound on the injured side, and pain when breathing.

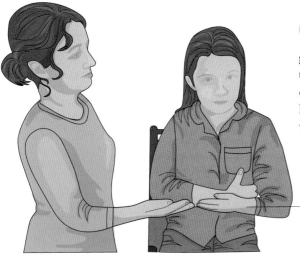

1 Help your child sit down and gently bring the arm on the injured side across her chest. Ask her to support her arm with her hand; you may need to help her.

Ask child to support arm on injured side

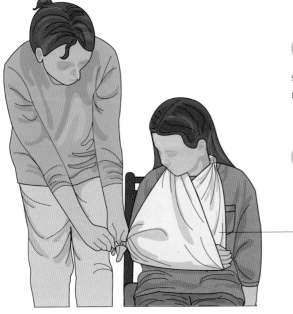

2 Support the arm on the injured side in an arm sling to minimize discomfort.

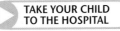
TAKE YOUR CHILD TO THE HOSPITAL

Support arm on injured side with a sling

! IMPORTANT

● **Do not** give the child anything to eat or drink because an anesthetic may be needed.

● **If** your child develops breathing difficulties, signs of internal bleeding, or shock, CALL 911 OR YOUR LOCAL EMS.

● **If** your child becomes unresponsive and has abnormal breathing, begin CPR immediately with 30 compressions. CALL 911 OR YOUR LOCAL EMS.

» see also

● Chest wound, p.50

● Internal bleeding, p.49

● Shock, p.36

● Triangular bandages, p.106

● Unresponsive child, pp.22–27

Arm injury

The treatment here is for injuries to the upper arm, forearm, and wrist. Move the arm as little as possible to minimize pain.

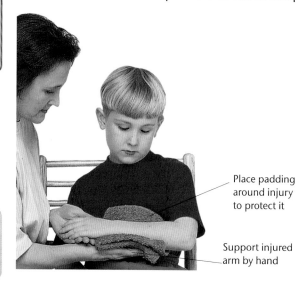

Place padding around injury to protect it

Support injured arm by hand

① Help your child sit down. Support the arm and encourage him to help. Place a soft pad around the injury and between his arm and his chest.

② For extra support place the arm in a sling and knot it on the uninjured side.

SEEK MEDICAL ADVICE

>> *see also*

● Collarbone injury, p.68

Elbow injury

Suspect an elbow injury if your child is unable to bend her arm, pain is increased by any attempts at movement, or there is swelling around the elbow. Keep the injury still because bone ends can damage blood vessels.

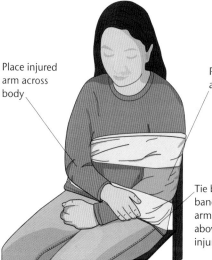

Place injured arm across body

Put soft padding around the joint

Tie broad-fold bandages around arm and body above and below injured elbow

① Help the child sit down, holding her arm across her body. Pad around the injury.

② Apply broad-fold bandages around the body and arm above and below the elbow. Check circulation at the wrist regularly.

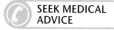

SEEK MEDICAL ADVICE

>> *see also*

● Check circulation, p.105

● Triangular bandages, p.106

Hand injury

This type of injury can be very painful. There may be several broken bones, and often a joint is dislocated. If your child's hand was crushed there may also be an open wound.

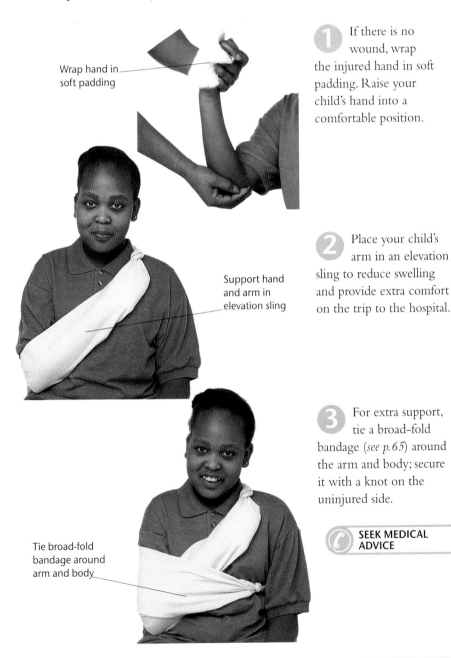

Wrap hand in soft padding

Support hand and arm in elevation sling

Tie broad-fold bandage around arm and body

1 If there is no wound, wrap the injured hand in soft padding. Raise your child's hand into a comfortable position.

2 Place your child's arm in an elevation sling to reduce swelling and provide extra comfort on the trip to the hospital.

3 For extra support, tie a broad-fold bandage (*see p.65*) around the arm and body; secure it with a knot on the uninjured side.

SEEK MEDICAL ADVICE

> **! IMPORTANT**
> ● If there is a wound, control the bleeding by pressing a clean dressing or pad over the site of the wound.

Jammed fingers

Hold the fingers under cold running water for a few minutes to relieve the pain and minimize swelling. If the fingers still hurt, apply a cold pack for 10 minutes (*see p.108*).

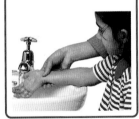

>> *see also*
● Crush injury, *p.49*
● Finger injury, *p.72*
● Severe bleeding, *p.38*
● Triangular bandages, *p.106*

Finger injury

Injury to a finger is common in children and can vary from simple cuts or abrasions to broken bones or tendon damage if, for example, the finger is shut in a door. It is important to get the injury checked because there are several blood vessels, tendons, and nerves in the finger that can be damaged, leading to deformity, bruising, and loss of sensation.

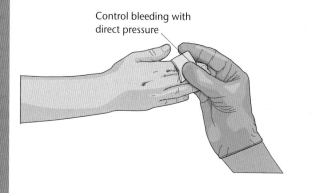

Control bleeding with direct pressure

1 Apply direct pressure over a sterile or clean pad to control any bleeding; do not press hard. Stop if this causes pain because there may be an underlying fracture.

2 Raise and support the finger, or ask your child to hold it up, to help relieve the pain and control the bleeding.

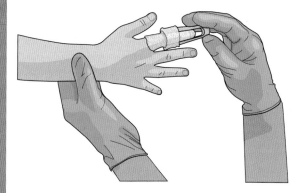

3 Secure the dressing with a bandage—a tube gauze bandage is ideal. For extra comfort, splint the finger to the next uninjured one.

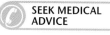

📞 **SEEK MEDICAL ADVICE**

OR

▶ **TAKE YOUR CHILD TO THE HOSPITAL**

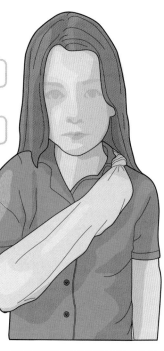

4 Support the arm in a raised position in an elevation sling if it makes your child more comfortable.

Apply elevation sling to help relieve pain

» see also

● Amputation, *p.48*

● Crush injury, *p.49*

● Severe bleeding, *p.38*

● Triangular bandages, *p.106*

Cramp

This is a painful muscle spasm that often affects the muscles in the foot, calf, or thigh. A cramp can occur after strenuous exercise or as a result of dehydration through excessive sweating. You can relieve the pain by stretching the affected muscles, then massage them to "relax" the spasm. Give your child water to drink to ease dehyration.

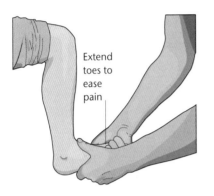

Extend toes to ease pain

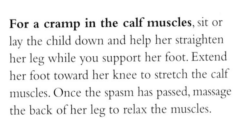

Extend toes to stretch toward shin

IMPORTANT

- **If** symptoms don't ease, SEEK MEDICAL ADVICE.

For a cramp in the foot, encourage your child to stand while you support the affected foot. Extend the toes upward to stretch the muscles. Once the spasm has passed, massage the underside of the foot with your fingers.

For a cramp in the calf muscles, sit or lay the child down and help her straighten her leg while you support her foot. Extend her foot toward her knee to stretch the calf muscles. Once the spasm has passed, massage the back of her leg to relax the muscles.

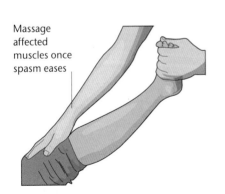

Massage affected muscles once spasm eases

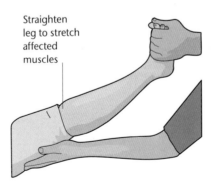

Straighten leg to stretch affected muscles

For a cramp in the front of the thigh, help your child lie down, then raise and support her leg. Bend her knee to stretch the muscles. Then, once the spasm has passed, massage the affected muscles.

For a cramp in the back of the thigh, raise and support her leg, and straighten her leg to stretch the muscles. Once the spasm has passed, massage the affected muscles.

see also
- Heat exhaustion, *p.88*

Bruises and swelling

Cold packs

Applying a cold pack to an injury helps minimize swelling and discomfort by reducing blood flow to the area. Make one by filling a plastic bag two-thirds full of ice and a small amount of water, or use a bag of frozen fruit or vegetables; wrap the bag in a cloth so that the ice does not make direct contact with the skin. You can also use cloth wrung out in cold water. (*see p.108*).

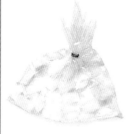

Leave a cold pack in place on an injury for 20 minutes, ideally uncovered.

After a fall or bump, bruising and swelling may develop rapidly. Resting, cooling, and raising the injury will minimize discomfort.

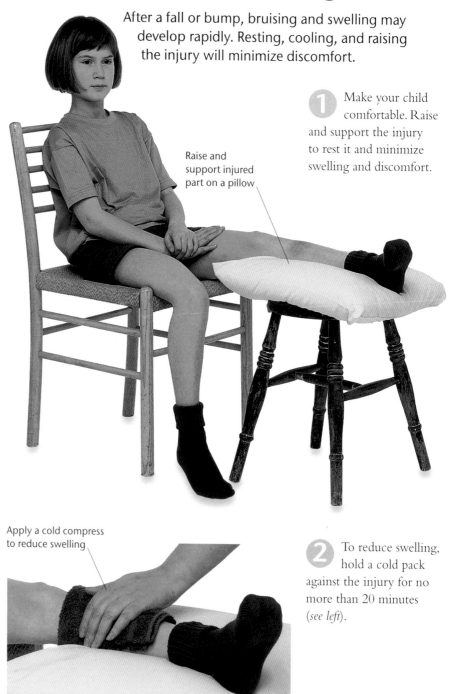

Raise and support injured part on a pillow

1 Make your child comfortable. Raise and support the injury to rest it and minimize swelling and discomfort.

Apply a cold compress to reduce swelling

2 To reduce swelling, hold a cold pack against the injury for no more than 20 minutes (*see left*).

Splinter

There is always a risk of infection with splinters. They are often dirty and the bacteria can be carried deep into the skin. Children are most likely to get splinters in their hands and knees because they crawl on the floor.

! IMPORTANT

- **If** your child is not immunized against tetanus infection, SEEK MEDICAL ADVICE.

- **Do not** poke at the area with a needle to remove the splinter.

- **If** you cannot remove the splinter, or if it breaks off, SEEK MEDICAL ADVICE.

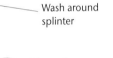

Wash around splinter

1 Clean the area around the splinter thoroughly with soap and warm water.

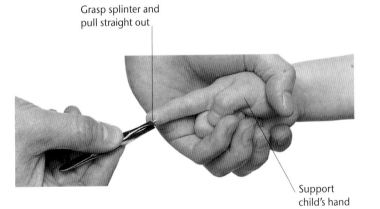

Grasp splinter and pull straight out

Support child's hand

2 Grasp the splinter as close to the skin as possible, and carefully draw it back out at the same angle it went in.

3 Clean the area again, washing well with soap and water.

≫ see also

- Infected wound, *p.42*
- Tetanus, *p.42*

Object in eye

Tiny hairs or specks of dust on the surface of the eye can be very uncomfortable for a child. Anything on the surface can generally be washed off easily; try to keep your child from rubbing her eye.

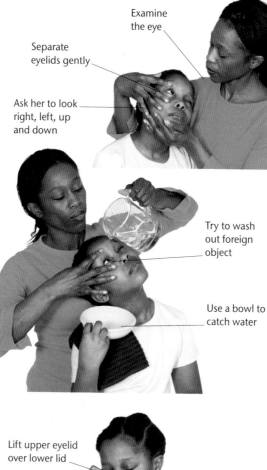

Examine the eye

Separate eyelids gently

Ask her to look right, left, up and down

Try to wash out foreign object

Use a bowl to catch water

Lift upper eyelid over lower lid

1 Help your child sit down, facing the light. Separate the eyelids of the affected eye. Ask her to look right, left, up, and down. Examine her eye thoroughly.

2 If you can see the foreign object on the surface of the eye, try to rinse it off using a pitcher of clean water. Tilt her head and aim for the inner corner so that water will wash over her eye. Or, try lifting it off with a damp swab or the corner of a handkerchief.

3 If an object is under the eyelid, you can ask an older child to clear it by lifting the upper eyelid over the lower one. You will need to do this for a toddler or young child; if necessary, wrap her in a towel first to stop her from grabbing your arms.

If an object has been removed

- **If** a hankerchief is used, be very careful not to scratch the surface of the eye.
- **If** eye is still red or sore TAKE HER TO THE OPHTHALMOLOGIST OR HOSPITAL.

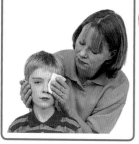

» *see also*
- Eyebrow or eyelid wounds, *p.44*

Object in ear

Children often push things into their ears. A hard object may become stuck, which can cause pain and mechanical hearing loss, which will be resolved when it is removed; it may even damage the child's eardrum.

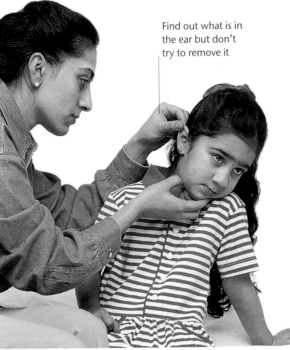

Find out what is in the ear but don't try to remove it

Reassure your child and ask her what she put into her ear. Don't try to remove the object, even if you can see it.

▶ **TAKE YOUR CHILD TO A DOCTOR, AN EAR DOCTOR, OR THE HOSPITAL**

If there is an insect in the ear

If an insect flies or crawls into your child's ear she may be very alarmed.

1 Help her sit down. Support her head with the affected ear uppermost.

2 Gently flood the ear with tepid water so that the insect floats out.

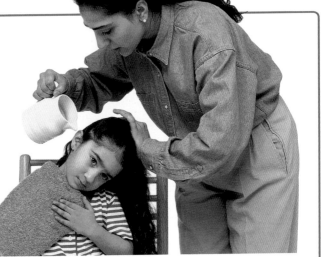

Object in nose

If your child has something stuck in his nose, his breathing may be difficult or noisy and his nose may be swollen. Smelly or blood-stained discharge from the nose indicates an object has been present for a while.

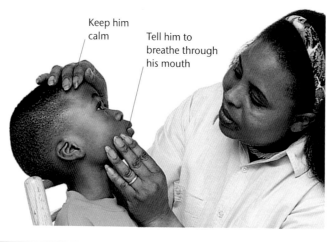

Keep him calm

Tell him to breathe through his mouth

1 Reassure your child and try to find out what he put in his nose. Tell him not to touch it.

2 Tell your child to breathe through his mouth until the object is removed.

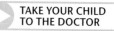
TAKE YOUR CHILD TO THE DOCTOR

Swallowed object

Young children often put small objects in their mouths and may swallow them. Most objects will pass straight through the digestive system. Small button batteries are dangerous because they contain corrosive chemicals. If you have any doubt about what your child swallowed and how to treat it, call the Poison Control Center (800-222-1222).

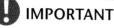

Ask him what he has swallowed

1 Reassure your child. Try to find out what the child has swallowed.

2 If the object is small and smooth like a pebble or a coin, there is little danger.

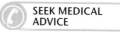
SEEK MEDICAL ADVICE

Animal and human bites

The main risk with any bite is infection; sharp pointed teeth can carry germs through the skin and into the tissues. Severe wounds with torn edges may need advanced medical care. Rabies is rare but possible; teach your child to watch out for wild animals and pets behaving strangely.

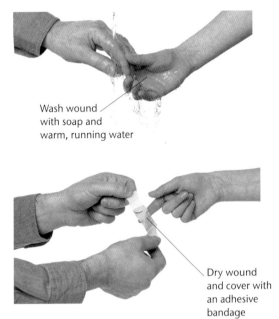

Wash wound with soap and warm, running water

1 Wash the wound thoroughly, using soap and warm water. Rinse the wound under running water for at least five minutes to wash away any dirt.

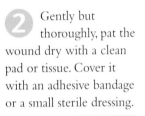

Dry wound and cover with an adhesive bandage

2 Gently but thoroughly, pat the wound dry with a clean pad or tissue. Cover it with an adhesive bandage or a small sterile dressing.

SEEK MEDICAL ADVICE

! IMPORTANT

- **If** the bleeding is severe, treat it; then, if there are signs of shock, CALL 911 OR YOUR LOCAL EMS.

- **If** you think your child may have been bitten by a rabid animal, take him to the hospital immediately.

- **Make** sure child's tetanus immunization is up to date.

» see also
- Severe bleeding, *p.38*
- Infected wound, *p.42*
- Shock, *p.36*

For a serious animal bite

1 If bleeding is severe, apply direct pressure over the wound, preferably over a sterile dressing or clean, nonfluffy pad.

CALL 911 OR YOUR LOCAL EMS

2 Cover the wound with a sterile dressing or pad and bandage firmly in place to help maintain direct pressure; make sure the bandage is not too tight (*see p.105*). Treat child for shock if necessary. Monitor the child's breathing, pulse, and level of reponse while waiting for help to arrive.

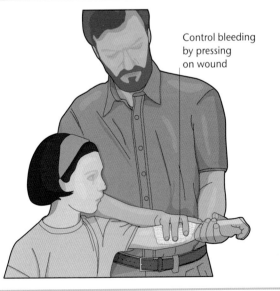

Control bleeding by pressing on wound

Insect sting

Bee, wasp, or hornet stings can be very alarming for a child, but they are rarely dangerous. Your child will experience a sharp pain followed by soreness, red skin, and slight swelling around the site of the sting.

If sting is in mouth

Give your child an ice cube to suck or cold water to sip and SEEK MEDICAL ADVICE. If swelling develops, CALL 911 OR YOUR LOCAL EMS.

» see also

• Anaphylactic shock, p.91

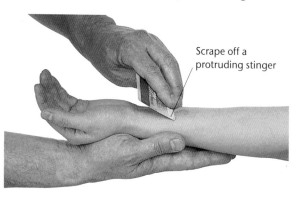

Scrape off a protruding stinger

Place a cold pack over area

1 If the stinger is still in the skin, brush or scrape it off sideways with your fingernail or a plastic card. Don't try to remove it with tweezers because you may inject more venom into your child.

2 Place a cold pack (p.108) on the site for about 20 minutes to minimize the pain and swelling. Rest the injured part. If pain and swelling persist,

SEEK MEDICAL ADVICE

Poison ivy rash

If your child brushes against poison ivy, he may develop a blotchy, red, itchy rash that may frighten him. Reassure him and soothe the rash.

» see also

• Allergy, p.90
• Cold pack, p.108

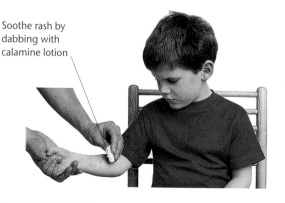

Soothe rash by dabbing with calamine lotion

1 To relieve the itching, dab the rash with cotton soaked in calamine lotion.

2 Alternatively, place a cold pack over the rash until the pain is relieved, about 20 minutes.

Tick bite

Found in woodlands and long grass, ticks are minute, spiderlike creatures that carry viruses and bacteria, including Borrelia, which causes Lyme disease. They attach themselves to people and animals to suck blood and can swell up to the size of a watermelon seed. Always check yourself and your child after walking in areas where ticks are likely to be found.

1 Using fine-toothed tweezers, grasp the tick as close to the child's skin as possible. Pull the tick's "head" upward using steady pressure. Don't twist or crush the tick because this can leave mouth parts (and saliva) embedded in the child.

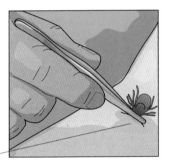

Grasp head as close to skin as possible

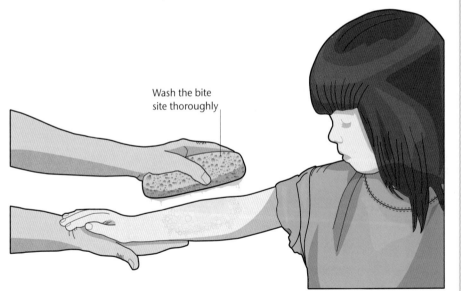

Wash the bite site thoroughly

2 Wash the area around the bite with soap and water.

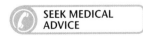
SEEK MEDICAL ADVICE

3 Put the tick into a sealed plastic bag and take it to your doctor, who may want to check that it is complete as well as test it for the bacteria that cause Lyme disease.

4 If your child develops a rash around the bite site or they start to display any flulike symptoms, *see box right*, seek urgent medical advice.

IMPORTANT

● **Do not** attempt to burn the tick or cover it with petroleum jelly in your attempt to remove it. You could injure the child and it may cause the tick to regurgitate infective fluid into her.

● **If** you can't remove the tick or you think mouth parts remain, SEEK URGENT MEDICAL ADVICE.

Lyme disease

The first sign of this may be a circular rash at the site of the bite that can develop up to 30 days later. The rash is described as looking like a bull's-eye. In many cases, however, this rash never appears, so if there are any other symptoms, such as fever or joint aches, SEEK URGENT MEDICAL ADVICE.

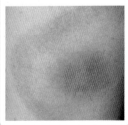

» *see also*
● Fever p.94

IMPORTANT

● **If** the sting is caused by Portuguese man o'war, immerse the area in hot water (104°F/40°C) for 10 minutes and SEEK MEDICAL ADVICE.

● **If** the skin is very red and painful, TAKE HER TO THE HOSPITAL.

● **If** the injury is extensive or your child develops anaphylactic shock, CALL 911 OR YOUR LOCAL EMS.

see also

● Anaphylactic shock, p.91

● Checking vital signs, p.14

Jellyfish sting

Jellyfish and sea anemone venom is contained in stinging cells that stick to a child's skin. Stings from marine creatures in temperate waters may not be dangerous, but those in tropical waters can cause severe poisoning. Vinegar or seawater should be used to flush the stung area.

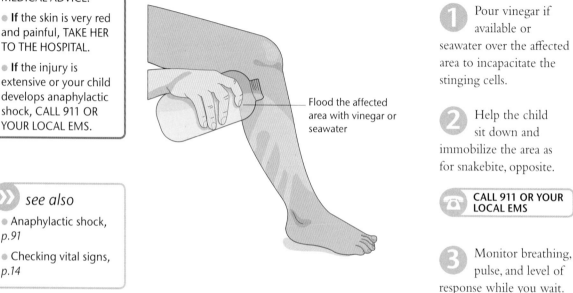

Flood the affected area with vinegar or seawater

1 Pour vinegar if available or seawater over the affected area to incapacitate the stinging cells.

2 Help the child sit down and immobilize the area as for snakebite, opposite.

CALL 911 OR YOUR LOCAL EMS

3 Monitor breathing, pulse, and level of response while you wait.

IMPORTANT

● **Make** sure the water is not too hot.

● **If** any spines remain embedded in the skin, or the foot starts to swell, elevate the limb and TAKE YOUR CHILD TO THE HOSPITAL

Marine puncture wound

When stepped on, the spines from a marine creatures such as catfish, lionfish, stonefish, and stingrays can puncture the skin, causing painful swelling and soreness. The spines can also break off and become embedded in a child's foot.

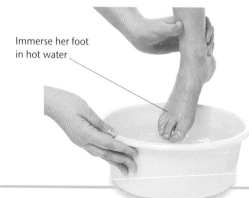

Immerse her foot in hot water

Immerse the injury in water as hot as your child can bear for about 30 minutes. Add more hot water as it cools, but be careful not to scald her.

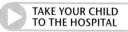
TAKE YOUR CHILD TO THE HOSPITAL

Snakebite

The toxin in a snake's venom can be either hemotoxic or neurotoxic. Hemotoxic venoms cause bruising, swelling, and bleeding, while neurotoxins can cause tingling, numbness, oral swelling, and also difficulty breathing.

☎ **CALL 911 OR YOUR LOCAL EMS**

1 Remain calm. Help the child lie down and stay still.

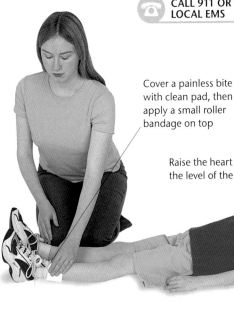

Cover a painless bite with clean pad, then apply a small roller bandage on top

Raise the heart above the level of the bite

2 Place a pad over the site and put a pressure bandage on top. Immobilize the bitten part with broad-fold bandages.

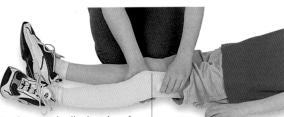

Apply second roller bandage from bite as far up leg as possible

3 If emergency help will be delayed, apply a second pressure bandage that extends from the bite as far up the limb as possible. You should be able to slip your finger under the bandage; loosen if necessary.

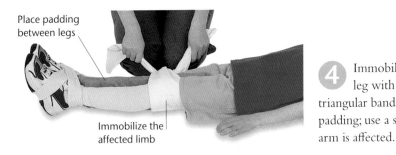

Place padding between legs

Immobilize the affected limb

4 Immobilize a leg with folded triangular bandages and padding; use a sling if the arm is affected.

❗ IMPORTANT

● **Do not** let your child walk around; keeping him still prevents the venom from spreading.

● **Do not** apply a tourniquet, cut out the wound, or try to suck out the venom.

● **If** possible, give an accurate description of the snake to the emergency services personnel, but never try to capture it.

● **If** your child develops a severe allergic reaction, treat as for anaphylactic shock.

● **If** your child becomes unresponsive and is not breathing normally, begin CPR immediately, with 30 compressions. CALL 911 OR YOUR LOCAL EMS.

》 see also

● Anaphylactic shock, p.91

● Checking vital signs, p.14

● Triangular bandages, p.65 and p.106

● Unresponsive baby, pp.19–21

● Unresponsive child, p.22–27

Hypothermia

This develops if the body temperature falls below 95°F (35°C), and if it falls further it is very serious. An older child is most likely to develop it outside in poor weather conditions, especially if there is a high wind-chill factor, or if a child falls into cold water. For babies, *see opposite*. If your child has had cold exposure and is shivering, she may have mild hypothermia. As she gets colder and the shivering stops, her condition is more serious. She may become listless, confused, or unresponsive.

For a child outside

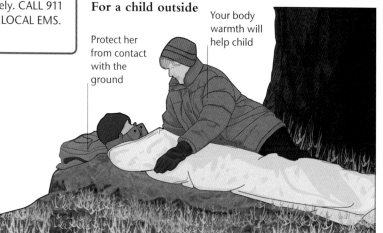

Protect her from contact with the ground

Your body warmth will help child

Take your child to a shelter. If there isn't one nearby lay her on a layer of dry insulating material such as soft brush or moss and protect her from the wind. Wrap her in a dry sleeping bag and a foil blanket if available. Use your body to keep her warm, too.

☎ **CALL 911 OR YOUR LOCAL EMS**

For a child indoors

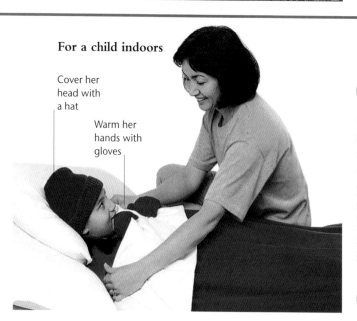

Cover her head with a hat

Warm her hands with gloves

1 If you can get to a shelter or your child is indoors, remove any wet clothes and replace them with dry ones. Cover her with plenty of blankets—you can put her in bed. Cover her head with a hat and make sure that the room is warm. Stay with her.

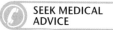 **SEEK MEDICAL ADVICE**

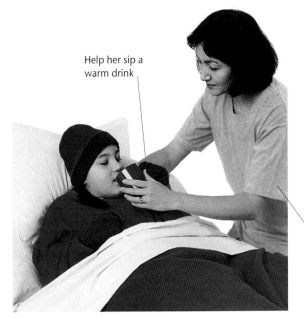

Help her sip a
warm drink

2 Give your child a
warm drink and
some high-energy foods,
such as chocolate.
Monitor her breathing,
pulse, temperature, and
level of response. Do
not leave her alone until
you are sure that her
temperature has returned
to normal.

Stay with her until
her temperature has
returned to normal

>> **see also**

● Checking vital signs,
p.14

● Unresponsive baby,
pp.19–21

● Unresponsive child,
p.22-27

Hypothermia in babies

A baby's temperature regulation is not fully
developed. He can lose body heat rapidly and
develop hypothermia in a cold room. Suspect
hypothermia if you are in a cool or cold
environment and your baby's skin feels cold; he is
limp and unusually quiet; and he refuses to feed.

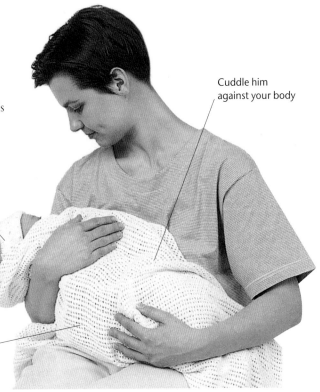

Cuddle him
against your body

Put a hat on
his head

Wrap him
up well

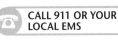 **CALL 911 OR YOUR
LOCAL EMS**

1 Rewarm a baby by
warming the room or
taking him to a warm room.
Wrap him in blankets.

2 Put a hat on his head
and cuddle him against
your body so that he is
warmed by your body heat.

Frostbite

If children are exposed to extreme weather conditions, the tissues of the fingers, toes, and other extremeties may freeze. Your child may have frostbite if she has pins and needles, with numbness and hard, stiff skin that is turning white and waxy. Shelter your child before treating her.

If the skin is broken

If there are any open wounds or the frozen skin is broken, cover the area with a soft gauze dressing and bandage it lightly in place. TAKE YOUR CHILD TO THE HOSPITAL.

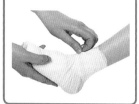

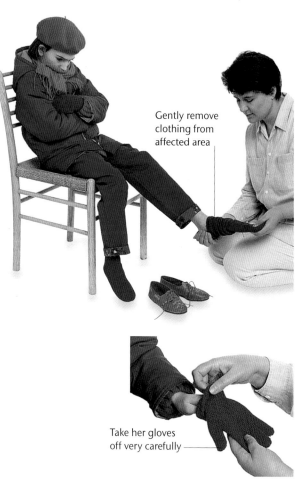

Gently remove clothing from affected area

Take her gloves off very carefully

1 While you are still outside, advise your child to put her hands under her armpits to use her body warmth to prevent her condition from worsening.

2 Once in a warm shelter, help her sit down, then start treatment. Gently remove constrictions from the affected area such as shoes, socks, and/or gloves and rings. Undo her coat. Start warming the affected area with your hands, in your lap, and/or in the child's armpits; don't rub them.

3 Place the affected part(s) in warm water—it should be around 104°F (40°C). Pat dry and cover with a light gauze bandage.

4 Raise the affected area to reduce swelling. Give your child the recommended dose of acetaminophen (not aspirin) to ease the pain.

▶ **TAKE YOUR CHILD TO THE HOSPITAL**

Sunburn

Sunburn is red, and may be itchy or tender. Babies and young children are very vulnerable: keep them in the shade; apply sunscreen; put on a hat, and cover with protective clothing in hot weather.

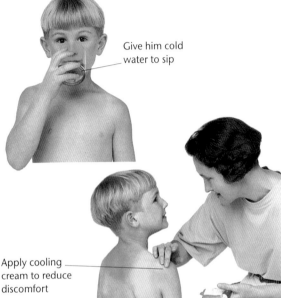

Give him cold water to sip

Apply cooling cream to reduce discomfort

1 Move your child into the shade or into a cool room and give him a cold drink. Cool the skin with cold water compresses.

2 Apply an aloe vera cream or gel to soothe the skin. Make sure you *know* your child is not allergic to it.

> **!** IMPORTANT
> ● If there is blistering or other skin damage, SEEK MEDICAL ADVICE.
> ● If your child is restless, flushed, dizzy, or has a temperature or headache, he may have heatstroke—CALL 911 OR YOUR LOCAL EMS.

> **»** *see also*
> ● Heat exhaustion, *p.88*
> ● Heatstroke, *p.89*

Heat rash

This is a prickly, red rash that develops particularly around the sweat glands on the chest and back and under the arms.

1 Help your child sit down in a cool room and undress her. Sponge the affected area with cool water.

2 Pat her almost dry with a soft towel, leaving the skin slightly damp. Apply calamine lotion if the rash itches.

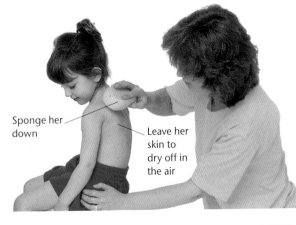

Sponge her down

Leave her skin to dry off in the air

> **!** IMPORTANT
> ● If your baby develops heat rash, remove some of her clothes to cool her, or bathe her in tepid water. Dry her gently, leaving her skin slightly damp.
> ● If the rash has not faded after 12 hours, or if she develops a raised temperature, SEEK MEDICAL ADVICE.

> **»** *see also*
> ● Heat exhaustion, *p.88*

! IMPORTANT

● If a baby or very young child develops heatstroke, undress him completely in a cool room.

● If your child becomes unresponsive and is not breathing normally, begin CPR with 30 chest compressions immediately. CALL 911 OR YOUR LOCAL EMS.

Heat exhaustion

Caused by excessive heat, whether the result of too many clothes or being left in a hot car, heat exhaustion can lead to dehydration—a loss of water and salts from the body because of excessive sweating without taking in fluids to replace what has been lost. A full, bounding pulse is a symptom.

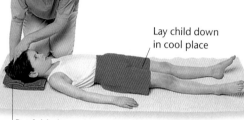

Lay child down in cool place

Put folded towel or cushion under head

1 Take your child into the shade or into a cool room. Help him to lie down.

Raise his legs

2 Raise and support your child's legs on some pillows. This improves blood supply to the brain. Encourage him to rest quietly.

3 Help your child sip as much cool water as he can manage. Later give oral rehydration salts or an isotonic sports drink to replace salt lost from the body.

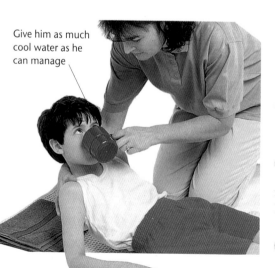

Give him as much cool water as he can manage

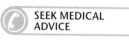
SEEK MEDICAL ADVICE

4 Monitor breathing, pulse, level of response, and temperature. If his condition worsens,

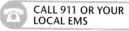
CALL 911 OR YOUR LOCAL EMS

›› see also

● Checking vital signs, p.14

● Heatstroke, opposite

● Unresponsive baby, pp.19–21

● Unresponsive child, p.22–27

Heatstroke

This is a life-threatening condition that develops if the body becomes overheated in hot surroundings. Treat your child for heatstroke if she develops a sudden headache; is confused; has hot, flushed, dry skin; is becoming unresponsive; and has a temperature of over 104°F (40°C). A rapidly weakening pulse is very serious.

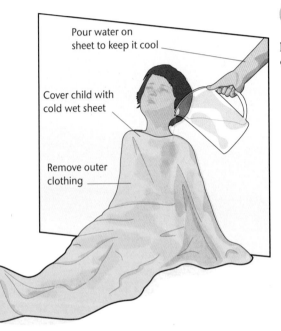

Pour water on sheet to keep it cool

Cover child with cold wet sheet

Remove outer clothing

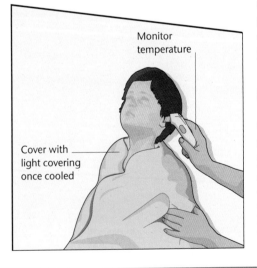

Monitor temperature

Cover with light covering once cooled

1 Quickly move child into a cool place. Remove as much outer clothing as you can.

CALL 911 OR YOUR LOCAL EMS

2 Help the child sit down on ground. Support her with pillows and/or against a wall and wrap her in a cold, wet sheet. Gently pour more water over the sheet to keep it cool.

3 A fan, and icepacks applied to the groin and armpits, will also help cool the child, but make sure she doesn't shiver, which will actually raise her core temperature.

4 Replace wet sheet with dry, light cover. Reassure your child and monitor breathing, pulse, level of response, and temperature while waiting for help to arrive. Repeat the cooling if her temperature starts to rise again.

! IMPORTANT

● **If** a baby or very young child develops heatstroke, undress him completely in a cool room.

● **If** your child becomes unresponsive and is not breathing normally, begin CPR with 30 chest compressions immediately. CALL 911 OR YOUR LOCAL EMS.

》》 see also

● Checking vital signs, *p.14*

● Unresponsive baby, *pp.19–21*

● Unresponsive child, *p.22–27*

Allergy

This is an abnormal reaction in the body's defenses that occurs in response to exposure to an allergen, and symptoms vary depending on the cause. Common allergens include pollen; dust; some foods such as nuts, shellfish, and eggs; as well as insect stings or bites. Mild allergy normally develops slowly, and a child may have an itchy rash or raised blotchy areas on his skin, sneezing, and red itchy eyes. Any swelling of the feet, hands, and/or face; wheezing; and even stomach pain, vomiting, and diarrhea can be signs of a serious anaphylactic reaction.

> **! IMPORTANT**
>
> ● **If the child's condition does not improve, the rash worsens or he develops breathing difficulties and/or swelling of the face or neck or is becoming distressed, treat for anaphylactic shock, *opposite*. CALL 911 OR YOUR LOCAL EMS.**

1 Try to identify the cause and try to remove the allergen from the child or the child from the allergen. If pollen is the allergen, move him indoors. If he has a reaction to laundry detergent, remove the affected clothing.

2 Treat any symptoms. For example, soothe an itchy rash with calamine lotion. Suggest he use his asthma medication if necessary.

3 Talk to your pharmacist because some mild allergies can be controlled with over-the-counter medication formulated for children. If the symptoms persist,

(SEEK MEDICAL ADVICE

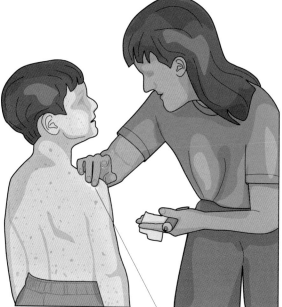

Dab calamine on itchy skin

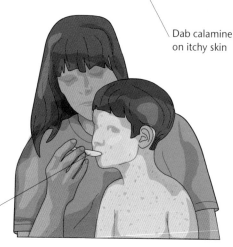

Offer recommended dose of antihistamine medication

> **» see also**
>
> ● Asthma, *p.35*
>
> ● Anaphylactic shock, *opposite*

Anaphylactic shock

This is a severe allergic reaction affecting the whole body that may develop within a few minutes of, for example, the injection of a drug, an insect sting, or ingestion of a food. It causes constriction of the air passages and swelling of the face and neck that can result in suffocation. Suspect anaphylactic shock if your child has increased difficulty breathing. Skin may be blotchy or flushed.

> **!** **IMPORTANT**
>
> • **If child has a known allergy and has her own medication, help her use it or give it to her yourself,** *see below.*
>
> • **If your child becomes unresponsive and is not breathing normally, begin CPR with 30 chest compressions immediately. CALL 911 OR YOUR LOCAL EMS**

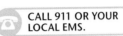 **CALL 911 OR YOUR LOCAL EMS.**

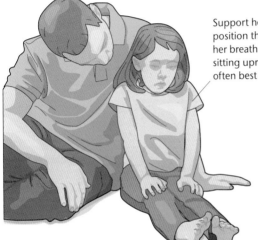

Support her in a position that helps her breathing; sitting upright is often best

1 Help your child into a position that helps breathing. Help with medication.

2 Monitor breathing, pulse, and level of response as you wait for emergency help. If pulse weakens and she becomes pale, treat for shock.

> **»** *see also*
>
> • Checking vital signs, *p.14*
> • Shock, *p.36*
> • Unresponsive baby, *pp.19–21*
> • Unresponsive child, *pp.22–27*

Administering an auto-injector

A child with a known allergy is often prescribed medication—usually an auto-injector of epinephrine—to use in the event of a reaction.

1 Hold the injector with your fist and remove the safety cap; don't put your thumb over the end.

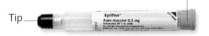

Tip

Safety cap

EpiPen®
Auto-Injector 0.3 mg

Push injector into thigh muscle (through clothing) until it clicks

2 Place the tip firmly against the child's thigh to release the medication. Hold it in place for 10 seconds, remove it, and rub the injection site for 10 seconds; repeat at 5-minute intervals if there's no improvement.

Diabetic emergency

If a child with Type 1 diabetes has low blood sugar he may be weak or hungry; confused or behaving aggressively; sweating; and very pale. He may also have a strong, pounding pulse and breathing may be shallow.

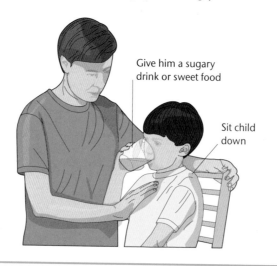

Give him a sugary drink or sweet food

Sit child down

Help your child to sit down and give him 0.5–0.7oz of glucose (5fl.oz orange juice, or 3tsp sugar) to raise his blood sugar levels. If he recovers, give him more. Check his glucose levels and monitor him until he is fully recovered.

SEEK MEDICAL ADVICE

If the child becomes unresponsive

If she is breathing, place her in the recovery position, p. 26. Then,

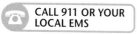
CALL 911 OR YOUR LOCAL EMS

1 If she is not breathing normally, begin CPR immediately (see p. 24) with 30 chest compressions.

2 Open airway and give 2 rescue breaths.

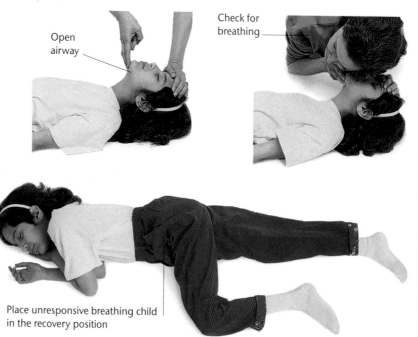

Open airway

Check for breathing

Place unresponsive breathing child in the recovery position

Fainting

Your child may be about to faint if she complains of feeling weak, sweaty, and nauseous, and is very pale. The period of unresponsiveness is brief and accompanied by a slow pulse; recovery is rapid and complete.

1 Help your child lie down and raise her legs above the level of her heart; this helps improve the blood flow to the vital organs. Support her legs on a pile of pillows or folded blankets.

2 Reassure your child and help her sit up gradually. If she starts to feel faint again, help her to lie back down until she feels better, then try again. If you are concerned about your child after the faint,

SEEK MEDICAL ADVICE

! IMPORTANT

● **Do not** sit your child on a chair with her head down if she is feeling faint because she may fall off and hurt herself.

● **If** your child becomes unresponsive and is not breathing normally, begin CPR immediately with 30 compressions. CALL 911 OR YOUR LOCAL EMS.

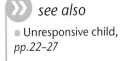

see also
● Unresponsive child, pp.22–27

Cool her by fanning her face

Raise her legs above the level of her heart

Fever

A body temperature that is above 100.4°F (38°C) indicates fever. An infection is the usual cause. A moderate fever is not harmful, but a temperature above 102.2°F (39°C) can be dangerous and may trigger seizures, particularly in very young children. As the fever advances she will have hot, flushed skin, be sweating, and have a headache.

> **!** **IMPORTANT**

- **If** your baby is under three months old, you should not give her acetaminophen syrup unless you are advised to do so by your doctor.

- **If** your child is very hot, take off as many clothes as possible; but do not sponge with water to cool her.

- **If** your child complains of a severe headache, suspect meningitis. TAKE YOUR CHILD TO THE HOSPITAL or CALL 911.

- **Raised** body temperature can be caused by overheating, *see* Heatstroke *p.89.*

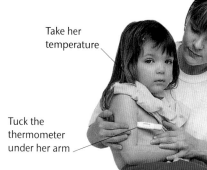

Take her temperature

Tuck the thermometer under her arm

Leave a drink beside her

>> *see also*

- Febrile seizures, *p.96*
- Heatstroke, *p.89*
- Meningitis, *opposite*

Give her the recommended dose of acetaminophen syrup

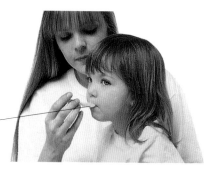

1 Take your child's temperature. If you are using a digital thermometer, on a young child lift your child's arm and tuck the pointed end into her armpit. Fold her arm over her chest and leave the thermometer in place until it beeps; an armpit reading will be about 1°F (0.5°C) lower than under the tongue.

2 Make your child comfortable on a bed or sofa, but do not cover her. To help bring down her temperature, make sure she has plenty of water or diluted fruit juice to drink.

3 You can give her the recommended dose of acetaminophen syrup (not aspirin) to help reduce her temperature; never give aspirin to anyone under the age of 16 years.

Meningitis

This is a life-threatening infection affecting the tissues that surround the brain. In the early stages your child will have a flulike illness with a high temperature. If his neck is stiff and his eyes are sensitive to light, he needs immediate medical evaluation. Take him to the hospital or call 911 or your local EMS. He may complain of cold hands and feet, or joint and limb pain. As infection develops he is likely to have a headache, begin vomiting, and become increasingly drowsy. Later, a red or purple rash may develop that does not disappear if pressed.

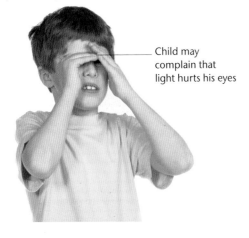

Child may complain that light hurts his eyes

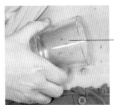

Meningitis rash will remain visible if you press a glass against it

Press side of a glass against the rash

! **IMPORTANT**

● **If** there is any delay contacting medical advice, or if you are concerned about your child's condition, TAKE YOUR CHILD TO THE HOSPITAL or CALL 911 even if you have already seen a doctor.

● **In** some cases, the rash may not develop, or if it does, it will be one of the last symptoms to appear.

1 If your child has a high fever and a flulike illness, monitor him carefully. If light hurts his eyes and he has a stiff neck, he needs immediate medical attention.

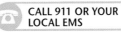
☎ **CALL 911 OR YOUR LOCAL EMS**

2 Treat fever. Give him plenty of fluids to drink and the recommended dose of acetaminophen syrup (not aspirin). Check your child's body for signs of a rash. If you see any spots, press a glass gently against them. If you can still see the spots through the glass,

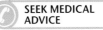
SEEK MEDICAL ADVICE

» *see also*
● Febrile seizures, *p.96*
● Fever, *opposite*

Febrile seizures

Young children may develop these seizures when they have a high temperature. Suspect a febrile seizure if your child has a fever and is having a seizure: she is shaking vigorously; flushed and sweating with a very hot forehead; eyes are rolled upward, fixed, or squinting; she is holding her breath and her face looks blue; she is clenching her fists.

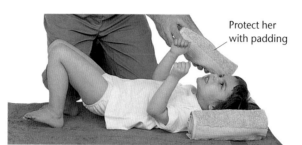

Protect her with padding

1 Place soft padding, such as towels or pillows, around your child so that even violent movement will not lead to injury.

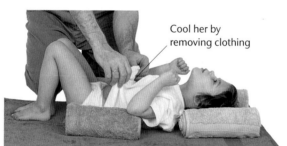

Cool her by removing clothing

2 Undress your child to help cool her down. Make sure there is a good supply of cool fresh air, but be careful not to overcool her.

After seizure stops, cover her with a sheet

Place her in recovery position

3 When the seizure stops, place her in the recovery position. Cover her with a light blanket or sheet and reassure her. If her temperature rises again, repeat steps 1 and 2.

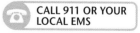 **CALL 911 OR YOUR LOCAL EMS**

>> see also

● Fever, *p.94*

● Unresponsive baby, *pp.19–21*

● Unresponsive child, *pp.22–27*

Epileptic seizures

These are caused by a disturbance in the electrical activity of the brain. A seizure may progress through stages: sudden loss of responsiveness, sometimes with a cry; rigidity and arching of back; breathing may cease; jerking or vigorous shaking movements begin; froth or bubbles appear at the mouth, possibly blood stained; loss of bladder or bowel control. The child will be responsive again within a few minutes and appear dazed. Afterward she may fall into a deep sleep.

Clear away nearby objects, such as chairs

1 If your child starts to fall, help her to the floor. Prevent injury by clearing away objects that she may knock against.

2 Place padding under or around her head to prevent injury.

3 When her seizure is over, your child may become unresponsive. Remove any padding and open her airway and check breathing.

Protect her head with soft padding —make sure it cannot cover airways

4 If she is breathing, place her in the recovery position. Stay with her until she is fully recovered. She may feel dazed and behave oddly, or sleep deeply.

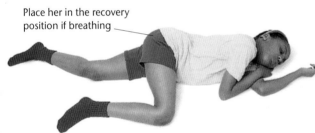

Place her in the recovery position if breathing

SEEK MEDICAL ADVICE

IMPORTANT

● **Do not** hold her down or try to move her during the seizure.

● **Do not** put anything in her mouth or give her anything to eat or drink.

● **Look** for a card or bracelet alerting you to the fact that a child has a history of epilepsy.

● **If** your child has never had a seizure before, it lasts more than 5 minutes, she has repeated seizures, or if she is unresponsive for more than 10 minutes, CALL 911 OR YOUR LOCAL EMS.

Absence seizures

These seizures can be recognized by a momentary "switching off," some facial twitching, or distracted movements such as lip-smacking. If this happens, reassure the child and seek medical advice.

see also

● Unresponsive baby, *pp.19–21*

● Unresponsive child, *pp.22–27*

! IMPORTANT

● **If** vomiting is prolonged, your child may need to be treated with oral rehydration solutions. SEEK MEDICAL ADVICE.

● **Do not** give your child antidiarrheal medication.

Vomiting and diarrhea

A baby or child who is suffering repeated vomiting and/or diarrhea can become dehydrated very quickly. It is important to replace lost fluids by giving your child sips of water. Don't give a baby or child milk unless you are breastfeeding.

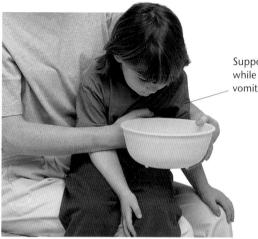

Support her while she vomits

1 If your child is vomiting, hold her over a bowl. Support her upper body with your free hand while she vomits. Reassure her.

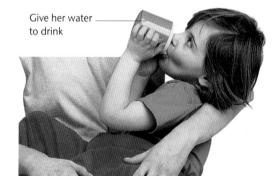

Give her water to drink

2 Give her drinks of water to replace any fluid loss and to remove the unpleasant taste. Encourage her to sip each drink slowly.

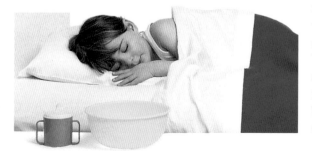

3 Let her rest quietly, in bed if she wants to. Make sure the bowl is still at hand in case she vomits again, and give a fresh drink of water. When she is hungry again, offer easily digested foods such as pasta, bread, or potatoes in the first 24 hours.

Stomachache

This is generally caused by a stomach upset, gas, constipation, or even stress.

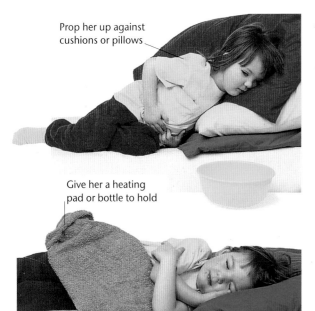

Prop her up against cushions or pillows

Give her a heating pad or bottle to hold

1 Make your child comfortable on a sofa or bed. Help her lie back against cushions or pillows. She may want to vomit, so leave a bowl near her.

2 Warmth may help relieve the pain. Give your child a heating pad to hold against her stomach. Avoid giving her anything to eat until pain subsides.

Appendicitis

Suspect appendicitis if your child complains of waves of pain in the middle of his abdomen or of acute pain either starting or settling in the right lower abdomen. He may also have a raised temperature, no appetite, nausea, vomiting, and diarrhea.

Suspected appendicitis must be treated promptly. Help your child lie down. Do not give him anything to eat or drink because he may need an anesthetic.

SEEK MEDICAL ADVICE

Pain may start here

Pain settles here

IMPORTANT

- **If** pain does not begin to subside, or if there is a discharge from the ear, fever, or hearing loss, SEEK MEDICAL ADVICE.

Pressure-change earache

This may happen on plane trips, particularly when taking off or landing, or when traveling through tunnels. To make the ears "pop" so that the pressure is relieved, an older child should close her mouth, hold her nose, and blow down it. Sucking a piece of hard candy may also help.

Earache

This is most commonly caused by an ear infection following a cold or flu. Earache can also be the result of a child putting something in her ear.

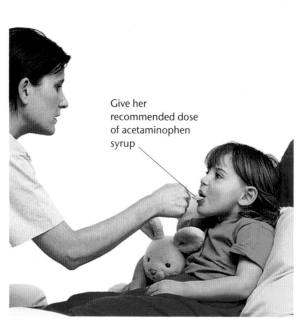

Give her recommended dose of acetaminophen syrup

1 Make your child comfortable. Help her sit up supported by pillows or cushions if lying down makes the earache worse. You can give the recommended dose of acetaminophen syrup or ibuprofen (not aspirin). Never give aspirin to anyone under the age of 16 years.

2 Applying heat may help soothe the pain. Prepare a covered hot water bottle and tell your child to lie down with her painful ear against it.

Provide a covered hot water bottle to place against her ear

Prop her up with pillows

Toothache

A toddler who complains of toothache may have a new tooth coming through. An older child may have tooth decay or an infection.

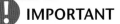

IMPORTANT
● **If** jaw is swollen and pain is severe, SEEK DENTAL ADVICE.

Give her recommended dose of acetaminophen syrup

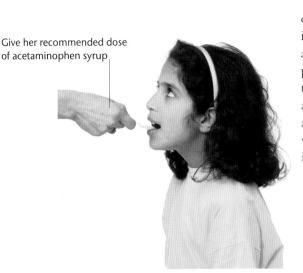

1 Give your child the recommended dose of acetaminophen or ibuprofen syrup (not aspirin) to relieve the pain. Never give asprin to anyone under the age of 16 years. Arrange an early appointment with your child's dentist if pain persists.

Give her a covered hot water bottle to lie against

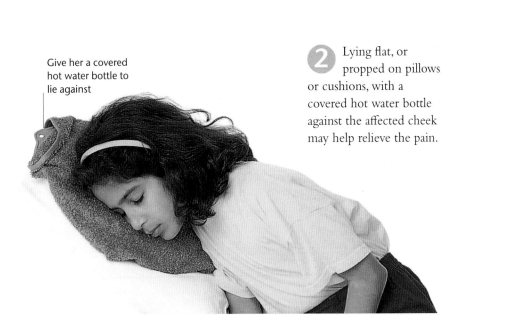

2 Lying flat, or propped on pillows or cushions, with a covered hot water bottle against the affected cheek may help relieve the pain.

A well-stocked first aid kit

- Disposable gloves (choose latex free)
- Small and large roller bandages
- Tube-gauze bandage
- Blunt-ended scissors
- Plastic tweezers
- Pack of gauze swabs
- Triangular bandages
- Tape for securing dressing pads and bandages—ideally hypoallergenic
- Sterile nonadhesive pads
- Adhesive bandages
- Sterile dressings

First aid kit

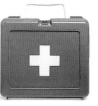

Keep first aid kits in your car and in your home. You can buy kits already made up. You may want to add extra dressings and bandages or specialized adhesive bandages—blister bandages, for example. Make sure the first aid box is readily accessible and easy to identify, and check the contents regularly. Do not keep medicines in the same box; they should be locked in a medicine cabinet. A well-stocked kit might contain the articles shown here. *See p.108 for alternative household items.*

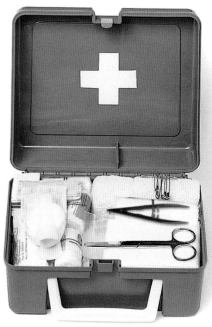

Blunt-ended scissors

Plastic tweezers

Dressings

Adhesive bandages (dressings) are used for minor wounds. Keep several different sizes and shapes, including a selection of larger sterile dressings for more serious wounds.

Adhesive bandages

Gauze swabs

Sterile nonadhesive pad

Sterile dressing with bandage attached

Bandages

Keep a variety of bandages to secure dressings and support injured joints. Conforming bandages shape themselves to the contours of the body and so are easy to use. Triangular bandages can be used as slings and for broad- and narrow-fold bandages.

Tape for securing dressings

Small conforming bandage

Large conforming bandage

Safety pins for securing bandages

Bandage clip

Tube-gauze finger bandage and applicator

Bandage slides over applicator

Folded triangular bandage

Additional useful equipment

- If you have a notepad and pen or pencil you can write down important information about a child's condition to give to the emergency services personnel.
- Keep a flashlight beside your home first aid kit (for use in the event of a power failure), and in your car; check the batteries regularly.
- Plastic face shields or face masks can protect you and a child from cross-infection when you are giving rescue breaths.
- Keep a plastic or foil emergency survival blanket or bag in your car.
- Always carry a warning triangle in your car and place it in the road behind the car in the event of a breakdown or crash.

ORAL REHYDRATION SALTS
Packets of rehydration salts are added to water. Use them to treat dehydration resulting from heat exhaustion or vomiting.

INSTANT ICE PACKS
Keep a pack of these in the car—they are especially useful when you do not have access to a freezer.

Digital thermometer

Ear thermometer

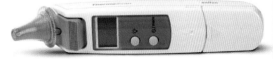

THERMOMETER
Choose one with an easy-to-read screen. Check the battery regularly.

Dressings

Covering a wound helps the blood-clotting process and prevents infection. Dressings should not be fluffy and must be large enough to cover the wound and area around it. Wash your hands before applying dressings and wear disposable gloves if possible. If blood soaks through a dressing, place another on top. Make sure bandages are not too tight (*see opposite*).

Adhesive bandages

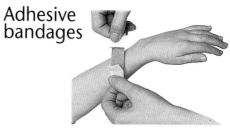

Remove wrapping and, holding the pad over the wound, peel back the protective strips. Press the ends and edges down.

Sterile pad

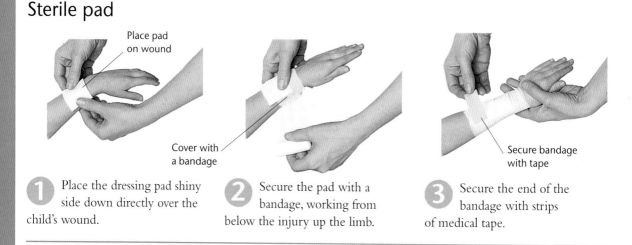

Place pad on wound

Cover with a bandage

Secure bandage with tape

1 Place the dressing pad shiny side down directly over the child's wound.

2 Secure the pad with a bandage, working from below the injury up the limb.

3 Secure the end of the bandage with strips of medical tape.

Sterile dressing with bandage

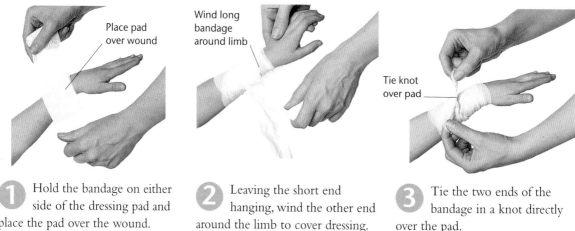

Place pad over wound

Wind long bandage around limb

Tie knot over pad

1 Hold the bandage on either side of the dressing pad and place the pad over the wound.

2 Leaving the short end hanging, wind the other end around the limb to cover dressing.

3 Tie the two ends of the bandage in a knot directly over the pad.

Bandaging

Use bandages to secure dressings, to help control bleeding, and to support injuries. Roller bandages can be used for any part of the body; conforming bandages are especially useful for bandaging joints or head wounds because they mold themselves to the shape of the body.

Check circulation

Do not apply a bandage too tightly—it will impair the circulation. To check, press on your child's nail or a patch of skin beyond the bandage, then release pressure. The color should return rapidly. If it does not, loosen the bandages.

Roller bandage

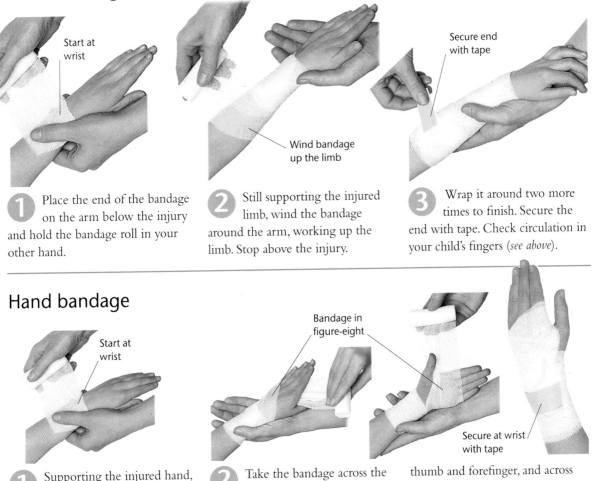

Start at wrist

Wind bandage up the limb

Secure end with tape

1 Place the end of the bandage on the arm below the injury and hold the bandage roll in your other hand.

2 Still supporting the injured limb, wind the bandage around the arm, working up the limb. Stop above the injury.

3 Wrap it around two more times to finish. Secure the end with tape. Check circulation in your child's fingers (*see above*).

Hand bandage

Start at wrist

Bandage in figure-eight

Secure at wrist with tape

1 Supporting the injured hand, hold the end of the bandage on the wrist and make two straight turns around the wrist.

2 Take the bandage across the back of the hand to the base of the little finger. Then take it around the palm, up between the thumb and forefinger, and across the back of the hand to the wrist. Repeat the figure-eight to cover the hand. Check circulation.

Triangular bandages

These are sold singly in sterile packs or can be made from a square of strong fabric folded diagonally in half. Triangular bandages are used for broad-fold and narrow-fold bandages (see p.65) or slings. Arm slings support injured arms or wrists, or take weight off an injured shoulder. Elevation slings are used to support hand injuries to minimize bleeding, pain, or swelling.

Arm sling

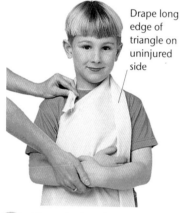

Drape long edge of triangle on uninjured side

1 Place the bandage between your child's arm and chest, easing one end up around the back of his neck on the injured side.

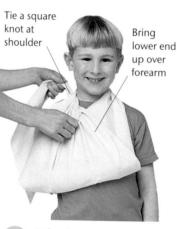

Tie a square knot at shoulder

Bring lower end up over forearm

2 Take the lower end of the bandage up over your child's forearm to the end at the shoulder and tie a knot just below the shoulder.

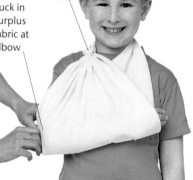

Make sure the knot is comfortable

Tuck in surplus fabric at elbow

3 Fold in the surplus fabric at the corner near the elbow and pin it to the bandage.

Improvised slings

If your child injures her shoulder, arm, or hand, you can make an improvised sling to support the injury until she receives medical treatment.

● Undo a coat or shirt button and tuck the hand of the injured arm inside the fastening, but don't use this method if the child's forearm or wrist is injured.

● Pin your child's sleeve up on the opposite side of his chest.

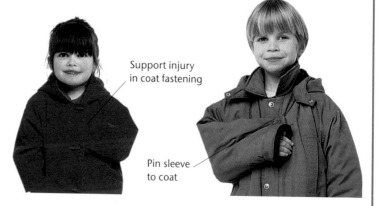

Support injury in coat fastening

Pin sleeve to coat

Elevation sling

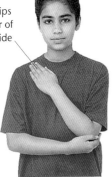

Rest fingertips on shoulder of uninjured side

1 Bring the arm on the injured side across your child's chest. Ask her to support her elbow.

Hold top corner at shoulder

Drape long edge across body

2 Lay bandage over child's arm, with longest edge on the uninjured side. Hold the top corner.

Scoop bandage up around elbow

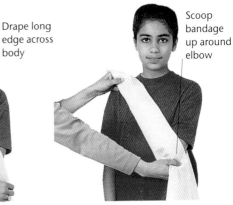

3 Support the child's arm and fold long edge of bandage in under injured arm.

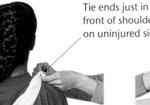

Tie ends just in front of shoulder on uninjured side

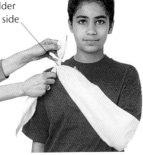

4 Bring the lower end up around her back, holding the elbow securely in the fabric. Tie a knot just below the shoulder and tuck the ends in.

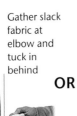

Gather slack fabric at elbow and tuck in behind

OR

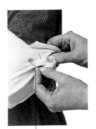

Pin slack fabric to front of sling

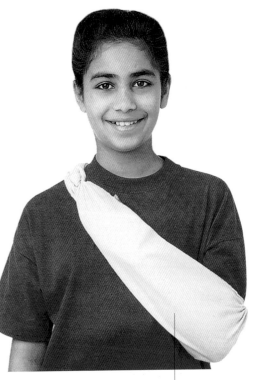

5 Secure the sling by twisting the excess fabric and tucking it in at the elbow or fold and pin in place.

Finished sling raises, immobilizes, and supports the injury.

Useful household items

You should keep a well-stocked first aid kit (*see p.102*) both at home and in the car. However, there are many everyday items around the home that are invaluable for first aid emergencies.

- Plastic credit cards can be used to scrape off an insect stinger (*see p.80*).
- A dish towel can be used as a pad to control bleeding or as an improvised dressing or to secure a dressing.
- Use vinegar to treat a jellyfish sting (*see p.82*)—it prevents the envenomation from getting worse and prevents pain from worsening.
- Cool or lukewarm water can be used to cool a burn if running water is not available (*see p.52*).
- Milk stops a knocked-out permanent tooth from drying out while you get the child to a dentist (*see p.47*).
- Use a thick book or wooden box as insulation when dealing with electrical injury (*see p.12*).

Making a cold pack

- Bags of frozen vegetables or fruit such as peas, corn, or blueberries make ideal ice packs because the bags mold to the shape of the body and stay cool for a long time. Wrap it in cloth before putting on your child for up to 20 minutes.
- Fill a sandwich or freezer bag two-thirds full of ice, then seal the bag; wrap it in cloth before putting on your child for 20 minutes.

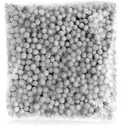

Frozen peas in a plastic bag

- Soak a washcloth in cold water, wring out excess water, then place it over the injury for 20 minutes.

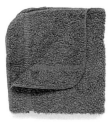

WASHCLOTH
Use a washcloth soaked in cold water to make a cold pack as well as to clean up a child after an incident.

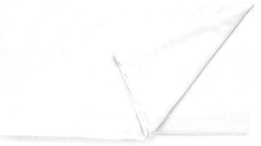

SHEETS AND PILLOWCASES
A clean cotton sheet or pillowcase makes an excellent loose protective covering for burns.

PLASTIC BAGS
A clean plastic bag can be put over a burned foot or hand and lightly secured with bandages or tape. Always cool the burn first.

PLASTIC WRAP
Cover cooled burns with plastic wrap to protect from infection.

Safety at home

Most incidents occur at home and over half involve children under the age of five. Many incidents are preventable if you:

- Plan the layout and position of objects and furniture at home with child safety in mind.
- Make sure that all windows are closed or inaccessible (don't leave chairs beside them).
- Never confuse containers by putting a dangerous substance, such as paint thinner, in a bottle that used to contain a harmless drink.
- Install smoke alarms, carbon monoxide alarms, fire guards, and safety gates in your home.
- Never pretend that medicines and pills are special candies to encourage a child to take medication. Keep all medicines locked away.
- Check for hazards when visiting friends and ask if you can move sharp or breakable objects.
- Teach your child basic safety rules.

Fire

If fire breaks out at home, it could be a matter of minutes before smoke overcomes you.

- Install smoke alarms throughout your home. If your home is on one level, install a detector between the living room and the bedrooms. If your house has two or more levels, install detectors at the foot of the stairs and on every floor outside the bedrooms; ideally they should be linked. If you live in an apartment building, there should be detectors in all communal areas too.
- Test smoke alarms regularly; replace batteries if they have them.
- Have an escape plan (*see p.11*). Make sure the whole family knows what to do if there is a fire, especially at night. Practice the fire drill with your children: shout "fire"; tell everyone to drop to the floor if there is smoke and crawl to the nearest exit from the rooms; shut each door behind you; arrange a meeting point outside where everyone should wait together. Don't go back for pets or treasured possessions.

Electricity

Protect your child from electric shock (*see p.12*) or fire caused by electric shorts.

- Cover outlets—put heavy furniture in front of them.
- Use bar-type fused adaptors with surge protectors on extension cords instead of block-type socket adaptors.
- Know where your fuse box is located, and how to change fuses in case one blows.
- Replace worn or damaged electrical cords.
- Coil trailing wires to prevent tripping hazards.
- Unplug electrical appliances at night, particularly the heaters and hairdryers.
- Keep power tools out of the reach of children.

Gas

Fit carbon monoxide alarms and have all boilers and gas appliances serviced regularly. Find out where your main gas valve is in case there is a leak. If you smell gas call 911 or the utility company:

- Don't turn lights or electric switches on or off—there may be a spark, which can cause an explosion.
- Don't light matches or cigarettes.
- Turn off the main gas valve and open the windows.

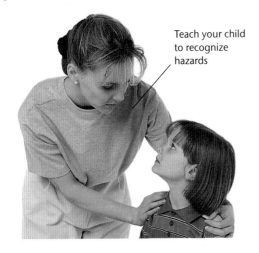

Teach your child to recognize hazards

Hall and stairs

The staircase is not a safe place for your child to play (*see below*).

- Make sure that toys are not left on the stairs for you to trip over.
- Put a light in your hall or on the landing so that your child can see if he gets up at night.

If you don't want the area too light, use a low-watt bulb. Never cover a lamp with a cloth because the cloth can easily catch fire.

- Don't let your child play on the landings or stairs of communal areas because the banisters may have large gaps between them.

Front and back doors

- Never leave your front door open.
- Don't let your child answer the door.
- Put the door catch out of reach of small children. If your toddler can reach the catch, install an additional bolt higher up the door and keep the door bolted.
- If the door has a dead-bolt that needs a key to open, make sure that the key is accessible to adults and older children so that they can escape if there's a fire.
- Install tempered or laminated glass in doors that have glass within 2ft 8in (80cm) of the floor. If this is not possible, put plastic safety film over it to prevent the glass from splintering if it is broken. Put stickers over the glass to make it more noticeable, especially for young children.

Floors

Tiled, polished, laminated, or rug-covered floors can be very slippery for toddlers and running children.

- Put nonslip liners under rugs.
- Keep hall floors free of toys and clutter.
- Check carpeting regularly for holes or loose carpet that might trip you or your toddler.

Stairs

A child is not coordinated enough to be able to walk downstairs safely until he is at least three years old.

- Fit safety gates at the foot of the stairs and across the upper landing or across your child's bedroom doorway (safety gates at the top of the stairs can be a trip hazard). The bars must be no more than 2⅜in

(5.5cm) apart, and avoid stair gates that open leaving a bar across the base because they are a trip hazard. Always open the gate; never climb over it; your child will copy you.

- Check your banisters regularly: the handrail and posts should be secured. Posts should not be too far apart—anything wider than 2½ in (6.5cm) apart should be boarded up. Don't let your child climb banisters. If the stairs or landing has horizontal rails (so-called ranch-type banisters), they should be boarded up because it is very easy for a child to climb them.
- Replace loose or worn carpet or steps. They are trip hazards.

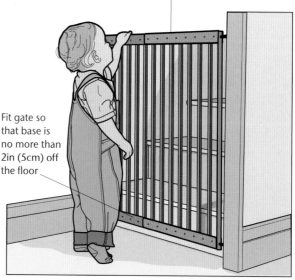

Keep the safety gate closed at all times

Fit gate so that base is no more than 2in (5cm) off the floor

Living room or family room

While your children are very young, try to arrange the room so that both children and your valuables are kept out of harm's way.

- If you have a balcony, ensure that it is too high for your child to climb. Block gaps in the railings with high-density fiberboard.
- Install safety glass in patio doors if the glass is within 2ft 8in (80cm) of the floor.

Carpets and curtains

- Check that there are no areas of carpet or rug that have holes or turned-up edges; either you or your child could trip.
- Wind up and tuck away all curtain ties and pull cords for blinds. Children can be strangled if they get caught in dangling cords.

Fireplaces and heaters

- Don't leave matches or lighters where your child can reach them.
- Cover all fires with a fireplace screen. Attach it to the wall to prevent your child from pulling it over. Also consider surrounding the hearth with a baby gate.
- Use a spark guard as well as a screen for open solid-fuel fires as an additional precaution.

Electrical equipment

- Attach wiring to the baseboards.
- Run long electrical cords behind furniture so that your child can't trip or pull on them.
- Replace items with worn wires.
- If your TV is on a stand, ensure that it is secure and cannot be pulled over. Ideally attach the TV to the wall.

Surfaces and furniture

- Place houseplants out of reach of young children. Dispose of any poisonous plants. Some can scratch or produce allergic reactions if touched.
- Do not place breakable or heavy objects on low tables. Set them well back from the edges of surfaces such as windowsills or mantelpieces.
- Put protectors on all sharp table corners, especially glass ones.
- Don't leave hot drinks, alcohol, glasses, cigarettes, matches, or lighters on low surfaces, such as coffee tables, where your child can reach them.
- Never leave a cigarette burning in an ashtray.
- Make sure all sofas and armchairs have a fire safety label; old foam furniture is lethal in a fire.
- Keep alcohol, firearms, and ammunition in a locked cabinet or safe.

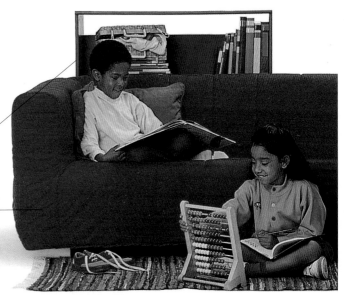

Ensure bookcases are secured to the wall

Sofas and armchairs must have fire-resistant fillings and coverings

Kitchen

This is the busiest part of your house, where you spend a lot of time with your children.

- Never hold baby or child in your arms when you are cooking or carrying a hot drink.

Doors

- Fit safety glass to any glass panels. Cover glass panels within 2 ft 6 in (80cm) of the floor with safety film, to keep glass from shattering or splintering if broken.
- Put some colorful stickers on the glass door panels to alert your child.

Floors

- Create a safe play area away from where you work. Don't let your child play between you and the work surface or anywhere you could trip over him.
- Avoid bumps and falls by wiping up spills immediately.
- Remove pet food bowls after use and keep that part of the floor scrupulously clean.
- Keep a box for storing toys and neatening clutter.

Garbage cans

- Discourage toddlers from rummaging in the garbage.
- Put sharp-edged cans and lids or broken glass straight into the outside garbage can.
- Keep the garbage can in a cabinet with a child-resistant safety catch.

> **! IMPORTANT**
>
> - Keep a fire blanket in the kitchen for smothering flare-ups. If you want to buy a fire extinguisher, consult your local fire department to find out which is the most appropriate type. Check the fire extinguisher regularly. For more on fires, *see p.11* and *p.109.*

Babies in the kitchen

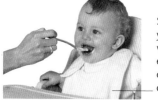

Stay with your child when he is eating in case he chokes

BOTTLES AND FOOD

- If your water is not safe due to microbes, sterilize all feeding equipment, or put it in a dishwasher.
- Don't leave a prepared feeding standing at room temperature, and don't keep the remains of the last feeding. Warmed and reheated feeds are breeding grounds for bacteria.

- Make fresh bottles for each feeding. Check the temperature before you feed your baby.

HIGHCHAIRS

- Always use the safety harness.
- Never leave the highchair where your baby can reach out and pull objects down from a surface.
- Never leave your child unattended in a highchair.

PLAY

- Put your baby in a playpen away from the cooking area, or put a gate across the doorway.
- Keep him out of range of any spills from the stovetop.

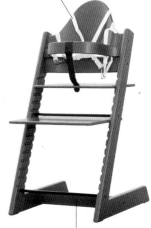

Attach a safety harness to the clips on either side of the chair

Choose a stable highchair with widely spaced legs

Tables and kitchen work surfaces

- Always be aware of your child's reach and keep all heavy, breakable, or sharp objects well back from the edges of work surfaces.
- Keep stools or chairs away from tables and work surfaces so that a young child cannot climb up.
- Tuck cords of electric food processors, toasters, blenders, and irons out of reach. Choose appliances with short or retractable cords if possible. It is not only the electricity from these appliances that poses a hazard; they can also cause deep cuts, burns, and crush injuries if a child pulls them off the counter.
- Leave all electrical appliances unplugged when they are not in use.
- Avoid using a tablecloth. It is tempting for a crawling baby or toddler to use it to pull himself up, bringing anything on the table down upon his head. Use placemats instead, or secure the cloth.
- Do not put your baby on a table or work surface when he is in a car seat—he could easily bounce himself off.

Cabinets and drawers

- Put safety catches on cabinets and drawers, particularly those containing matches, lighters, knives, scissors, and utensils; heavy pots, pans, or china; dried food, such as lentils or pasta, which may be a choking hazard; bottles containing alcohol; medicines; cleaning materials, such as laundry soap, or dishwasher detergent, even if fitted with "child-resistant" lids.

Refrigerators

Food poisoning can be caused by poor food storage. Take precautions to minimize risks:

- Keep cooked meat and poultry on a separate shelf from uncooked meat. Cover uncooked meat with plastic wrap.
- Don't store food in open cans; put leftovers into a clean container, cover, and put in the refrigerator.
- Check food regularly to see that nothing is kept beyond the "use-by" date.

Stovetops

Your child is obviously at risk of burns and scalds from hot oil or boiling water when you are preparing food.

- You can buy safety guards, but remember that a child can still poke fingers through some types and be burned by hot burners.
- Always keep your child away from oven doors; they can get very hot while the oven is in use and will stay hot for some time afterward. A crawling baby or toddler is particularly at risk. Try to teach your child what "hot" means so that he understands a warning.
- Keep ignition devices, matches, and lighters well out of reach in a cabinet fitted with a safety catch.

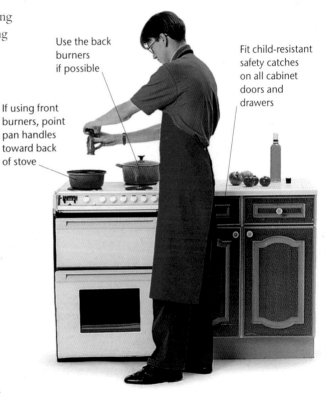

Use the back burners if possible

Fit child-resistant safety catches on all cabinet doors and drawers

If using front burners, point pan handles toward back of stove

Washers and dryers

- Keep small hands away from the glass door; it may get hot while the machine is on.
- Ensure that the door is closed when the machines are not in use. Your toddler may try to climb inside or even fill it with toys.

Bedrooms

The cabinets and drawers in bedrooms are always exciting places for toddlers and young children. Make sure any potentially hazardous items are out of reach because you may not always know when your child will decide to go exploring on his own.

Baby's cribs

- Make sure the crib is deep enough to prevent your baby from climbing out—at least 1ft 8in (50cm) from the top of the mattress to the top of the crib.

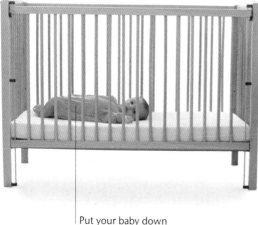

Put your baby down to sleep with her feet at the base of the crib

- Bar spaces must be between 1 and 2½in (2.5–6cm) wide to prevent your baby's head from being trapped.
- The mattress must fit the crib with a gap of less than 1½in (3cm) around the side or the baby's head could become trapped between the crib side and the mattress.
- Don't use a pillow for a baby under one year: it could suffocate him. If you need to raise his head, put a pillow under the mattress or raise one end of the crib.
- Use a sheet and cotton knit blankets rather than a quilt until your baby is one year old. Your baby could overheat or suffocate under a quilt.
- Don't put the crib near a heater or in a very sunny part of the room. Don't use a crib bumper.
- Put your baby to sleep on his back with his feet at the foot of the crib to lessen the risk of crib death; babies under 6 months should sleep in their parents' room.
- Remove toys from the crib as soon as your baby can sit up because he could use them to climb out.
- Once your child starts trying to climb out of the crib, transfer him to a bed.

Changing areas

- Keep all changing equipment in one place so that you never have to leave your baby alone on the changing mat. He will be safest on the floor, but if you have a changing table, remember that he might roll off if left even for a moment.
- Store diaper bags well out of the reach of babies because these present a suffocation risk.
- Do not have shelves above the changing area in case something falls off onto your child.
- Keep dangling mobiles out of his reach.
- Use a towel rather than talcum powder to dry your baby's skin because the fine particles can be harmful if your baby breathes in lots of them at once.

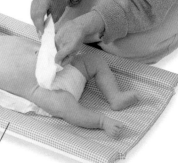

Change your baby on the floor on a changing mat so that he cannot fall

Children's bedrooms

This is a room where children are likely to be unsupervised, so it has to be as safe as possible.

- Ideally choose blinds without a loop mechanism, but if there is one attached to the blind, it must have a safety release that breaks under pressure. Stow curtain ties well out of reach of children.
- Don't use a bed guard when your toddler first moves to a bed; if you think he may fall out, put cushions on the floor beside the bed.
- A top bunk bed is not recommended for children under the age of six.
- Top bunk beds must have safety rails on both sides and any gaps in the railings or between the top of the mattress and the bottom of the safety rail should be no more than 2½–3in (6–7.5cm).
- Never let young children play on the top bunk.
- Remove toys from the floor by the bed at night.
- Make sure there are no wires near a child's bed.

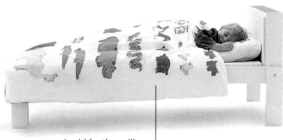

Avoid feather pillows and quilts because they can provoke allergies

WINDOWS

Make sure your child can't climb out of the window. In many areas, window guards are legally required for apartments with children under the age of 10.

- Install a safety catch, but make sure the window can be opened easily in the event of a fire.
- Don't place a piece of furniture below a window because it may encourage your child to climb up.

TOYS *(see also p.117)*

- Keep toys that are unsuitable for very young children separate from others. This way you can easily put them out of reach if your child is sharing a room with a younger child, or if you have young visitors.

Put nonslip liners under rugs

Your bedroom

Babies under 6 months should sleep in a crib in their parent's room—but not in a parent's bed.

- Perfume, hairspray, and makeup can be harmful if sprayed or rubbed in the eyes or swallowed, so keep them out of reach or in a drawer with a safety latch.
- Medicines and pills should never be left beside your bed, or on a dressing table. Put them out of sight and out of a child's reach, preferably in a locked cabinet.
- Scissors and sewing equipment should be kept in a drawer or cabinet with a safety latch.
- Never leave a mug, teacup, or a glass on the floor by your bed, especially at night. If your child happened to be in your bed, he could roll out onto the cup, mug, or glass.

Bathroom

Your child may be at risk from falls, drowning, scalding, or poisoning in the bathroom. Keep the door shut at all times to discourage him from going in. If you install a bolt on the door, attach it near the top of the door to prevent a young child from locking himself in.

Baths

- Check the temperature of the water before your child gets into the bath. Put your elbow in the water; if it is too hot for your elbow, it is too hot for your child. A child can be badly scalded by hot bathwater.
- Install an anti-scald device to regulate water temperature.
- Place nonslip mats in the tub and on the floor beside it.
- Keep babies and toddlers away from the tub faucets.
- Never leave a young child or baby alone in the bath (or in the care of another child). A baby can drown in just 1in (2.5cm) of water. If you need to answer the door or telephone, take your baby with you.

Showers

- Keep a constant check on the temperature of the water.
- Use nonslip mats in the shower and on the bathroom floor.
- Put safety film on a glass shower door so that glass is held in place in case of an incident.

Cabinets

- Store bathroom chemicals and other potential poisons, such as toilet cleaners and bleach, out of reach in a cabinet with a safety lock.
- Keep other hazards, such as makeup, aftershave, razors, nail scissors, and any medicines or glass containers, out of reach in a locked medicine cabinet.

Toilets

- Use a special child toilet seat adaptor and step for toddlers so that they can keep their balance more easily and feel more secure.
- Keep the toilet seat closed when not in use.
- Don't use block toilet cleaners that a young child could pull out and chew.
- Never use both toilet cleaners and bleach because the combination will produce toxic fumes.
- If your toddler uses a potty, keep it clean, but never leave bleach or cleaning agents inside it.

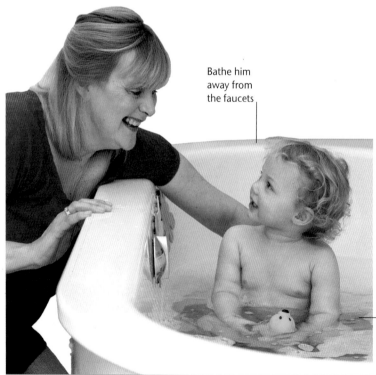

Bathe him away from the faucets

Use a nonslip mat in the bathtub

Toys and playthings

If you have children of different ages in your home, keep their toys in separate boxes. In particular, keep toys with small parts away from younger children.

Give your child nontoxic paints to play with

Choosing toys

- Buy toys that are appropriate for the age of your child, and buy from a reputable source.
- Don't give your child anything to play with that has sharp edges, or is made of thin, rigid plastic.
- Give him nontoxic paints or crayons.
- Don't buy your child old toys: they may be broken or covered in paint containing lead.
  - Avoid novelty toys that are not designed to be played with by young children: look out for warnings on the packaging.

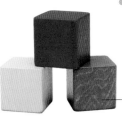

Check sets of building blocks for small pieces that could be a choking hazard for a younger child

Caring for toys

- Check toys regularly and always throw away any broken ones.
- Don't mix old and new batteries. Change them all at the same time; otherwise, the strong batteries will make the weak ones very hot.
- Keep toys in a toy box. Toys can bring about accidents or injuries if left on the floor.

Babies and toddlers

- Remove ribbons from a baby's soft toys.
- Check that the eyes, noses, ears, or bells on soft toys and dolls are well secured.
- Attach crib toys with a very short string and remove them as soon as your baby can sit up.
- Remove activity centers or bulky toys from a crib as soon as your child can stand because they provide a foothold for climbing out of the crib.
- Don't let babies chew on furry toys: the fur is a choking hazard.
- Never let a young child play with a toy that is not recommended for his age group: it may contain small pieces on which he could choke.
- Don't leave a baby or toddler to play in a room on his own.
- Baby push toys can help mobility and balance, but avoid "baby walkers," which are dangerous and may actually interfere with proper development and delay walking.

Make sure that toys that increase mobility are stable

Yard

Your yard can be a safe and interesting place for your children to play. Children will find their own corners to play in, but you must clear away trash and remove obvious hazards:

- Lock gates that lead out of the yard and make sure that fences are secure.
- Check garden furniture or play equipment regularly to make sure that it is safe. Place it over grass, not paving stones.
- Keep pets away from children's play areas.
- Make sure paving is even and remove moss so that neither you nor your child trip or slip.

Plants

Many plants are poisonous if eaten and digested in large quantities. Small pieces, or one or two berries, are not fatal but may cause some discomfort and stomach upset.

- Tell your child about the dangers of eating berries, and keep babies and toddlers away from them.
- Remove plants that you know to be poisonous, such as deadly nightshade, yew, and toadstools.
- Cut back any prickly plants, such as roses, brambles, and holly. They can give painful scratches, especially to your or your child's eyes.

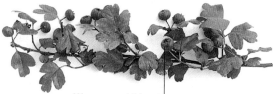

Warn your child not to eat berries or leaves

Sheds and bins

Sheds are inevitably used for storing chemicals and tools, and so are a potential hazard.

- Tell your child that the shed is out of bounds, keep it locked at all times, and hide the key.
- Put chemicals, such as weedkiller or slug pellets, out of reach in containers with child-resistant caps.
- Keep wheeled trash cans hinge side outward so that a child can't open them and climb in.

Water in the garden

Babies and toddlers are especially at risk if they slip and fall, even in shallow water. Maintain fencing to prevent children from entering a neighbor's yard where a swimming pool or pond may be a hazard.

- Never leave children unattended when they are playing in, or near, water.
- Keep ponds covered and fenced off, and cover rain barrels and empty trash cans that collect rainwater.
- Always empty out a wading pool when your children have finished playing in it and turn it upside-down in case it rains.

Gardening

- Don't put down chemicals when children will be playing in the garden.
- Don't mow the lawn while children are close by because stone chips may become dislodged and fly up into their eyes.
- Put away all garden tools when you have finished using them.

Check that he is playing in a clean, safe area with safe toys

Garage and car safety

Always leave your garage locked; likewise, keep the car locked, even if it is on a driveway off the road or in a garage. Keep the car keys where the children cannot reach them. Don't give the keys to your baby to play with because they are not clean and he could drop them.

Garages and driveways

- Keep the garage locked and discourage your child from going in there.
- Keep equipment, chemicals, or tools out of your child's reach and locked away if possible.
- Make sure you know where your child is when you are driving into, or out of, the garage or a drive.
- If you keep a chest freezer in the garage, it should be locked at all times.

Cars

- Never leave a young child unattended in a car, even if you can see the car.
- Don't let your child play with the car windows, whether manual or electric. Windows can trap a child's head or fingers.
- Remove the cigarette lighter from the car altogether.
- Watch out for your child's fingers when you shut the car doors.
- Use child locks on rear doors until your child is at least six years old.
- Teach your child to get out on the curb side.
- If your child is helping you wash the car, make sure you have removed the car keys from the ignition first.

Car seats

Always put your child in a special safety seat when you strap him into the car. The law requires that all children up to about 4ft 5in (135cm) traveling in cars use a child restraint—in some states this limit is 4ft 9in (144cm). Never carry a baby or child on your lap even in your seatbelt—it is not only dangerous (your baby could be thrown out of the car or crushed by your body weight in a crash) but it is also illegal.

There are various types of car seats—the correct one will depend on the age and size of your baby or child and your car. Ideally when you buy a seat, go to a retailer who will show you how to use it properly. Fit the seat exactly as the instructions describe. Most cars now have special Isofix seat fixings, which are more secure than seat belts, for child car seats, and connectors on the seats clip onto these fixings. Check that your chosen seat is approved for use in your particular vehicle. Then choose the correct seat for the weight and development of your child:

- Babies and toddlers up to 29lb (13kg) should travel in a rear-facing car seat. The safest place for your baby to travel is in the rear seat of your car. Do not place your baby in a rear-facing car seat on the front passenger seat if there is an airbag installed that cannot be disabled—the impact of an airbag inflating could cause serious injury.
- Older toddlers who have outgrown the height and weight limitations of their rear-facing seat (up to 40lb/18kg) need a front-facing car seat in the back seat of the car. Some seats have an integral harness for the child, which fits over his shoulders, across his hips, and between his legs. The seats are held in place by the Isofix fixings or an adult seat belt.
- Children who weigh more than 48lbs (22kg) can travel in a booster seat. Without them, adult seat belts are neither comfortable nor safe: the shoulder part cuts across the child's neck, and the lap strap lies across his stomach, which could cause internal injury in a crash. A lap strap alone is not sufficient because it does not restrain the child's upper body.

Finally, use a seat on every journey in a car, no matter how short—even in taxis.

Out and about

After the home, most childhood incidents occur in the street or in play areas. Teach your child the rules of the road from an early age, reminding him to stay alert for traffic and to cross in a safe place. It takes a long time for children to develop a true road sense.

What a child understands

- Three-year-olds can learn that the sidewalk is safe and the road is dangerous.
- Five-year-olds can learn how to cross the road, but they are still not able to put this knowledge into practice on their own.
- Eight-year-olds can cross quiet streets on their own, but they are not yet able to judge the speed and distance of traffic.
- Twelve-year-olds can judge the speed of an oncoming car, but are still easily distracted by friends.

Street and road safety

Whenever you are out with your child, show him how to be aware of his own safety.

- When out shopping or walking near a road, carry your toddler or keep him in a stroller to keep him from running off without you.
- Encourage a young child to hold your hand when you are near the road or waiting to cross a road.

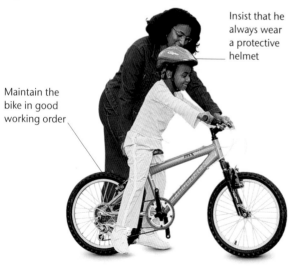

Maintain the bike in good working order

Insist that he always wear a protective helmet

Learning how to cross the road

Teach your child the rules of the road:

- Find a safe place to cross, then stop.
- Stand on the sidewalk, near the curb.
- Look both ways for traffic, and listen.
- If traffic is coming, let it pass.
- When there is no traffic near, walk straight across the road.
- Look and listen for traffic while you cross.

- Teach your child by example and always find a safe place to cross a road. This may be a crosswalk, a pedestrian crossing with lights, an underpass, or a footbridge. If there is no designated crossing point, aim for a large gap between parked cars, where you and your child can see a long way in both directions.
- At a crosswalk, teach your child to stop and wait until all the traffic has stopped and to stop at the island halfway across, if there is one.
- When using a pedestrian crossing with traffic lights, encourage your child to press the button and always wait until the traffic has stopped before crossing.

Bikes

- All children should wear a helmet when riding a bike.
- Children under 10 years old should not bicycle on roads in traffic without an adult, and all children should have training before going on the road.
- Make sure your child can be seen when he's riding his bike—with bright fluorescent colors by day and reflectors on his clothes and bike by night.

Where to play

What may seem common sense to you is not obvious to children.

- Show your child where it is safe to play—the playground, or local recreation area, for example—and supervise him if necessary.
- Teach your child the dangers of playing in open areas, such as roads, building sites, and quarries.
- Tell your child not to play in the street, or on pavement near the curb—even if your street is quiet.
- Tell him that he must never chase a ball, a pet, or another child into the road.

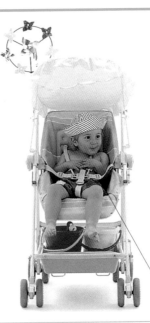

Harness your baby
into his stroller

Carriages and strollers

- Never push a carriage or stroller out into the traffic to see if the road is clear to cross. Pull the stroller to one side and check whether the road is safe. Remember that a child's stroller sticks out in front of you by at least 3ft (1m).
- When you park a carriage or stroller, put on the brakes and point it away from traffic.
- Never tie your dog to the stroller.
- Never leave a baby unattended.
- Keep your child away from the stroller when you are assembling or folding it to keep little fingers from being trapped.

On the playground

All playgrounds should comply with safety standards; report any faulty equipment in community playgrounds to your local authority.

- The play area must be safely fenced off and away from roads.
- There should be a soft, even surface, such as mulch or rubber tiles, around equipment.
- Slides should be no higher than 8ft (2.4m) and preferably constructed on an earth mound to break any falls.
- Carousels should be low, with a smooth surface, designed so that young children can't get their feet stuck underneath.
- Climbing frames should be no higher than 8ft (2.4m), completely stable, and built over sand or a very soft surface to break falls.
- Swings should set away from main play equipment.
- There should be a clearly defined play area for toddlers and young children, set away from the more boisterous activities of older children.
- There should be someone to contact if any of the equipment is faulty.
- Dogs must not be allowed inside playgrounds.

Put a young child in a swing with a safety guard and stay with him at all times

! IMPORTANT

- **Remind** your child of the dangers of talking to strangers. Have a code word that a friend can use if picking up your child. Tell your child not to go with anybody unless they use the code.

Traveling with babies and children

Away from your home all the same rules of safety apply. However, you should be aware that the place you are staying might not necessarily have been planned with young children in mind.

- If there is a swimming pool, never leave your child unattended in or near the water and, if there is a fence around it, keep the gate shut.
- Take baby milk and/or food with you; your child may not like what is available locally.

Traveling abroad

- Make sure your child's immunizations are up to date. Some countries recommend additional vaccination, or antimalaria medication; ask when booking a trip.
- Don't forget to take the necessary paperwork; babies and children need their own passports. It is a good idea to keep a photocopy of each passport (yours as well) in a separate bag.
- If you are renting a car, always ask for child safety seats, or take your child's car seat with you.
- Make sure rented cars are equipped with sufficient safety restraints and check that they are in good condition (not worn) and working properly.
- Take insect repellent suitable for babies and young children because they are particularly susceptible to insect bites. Apply the repellent in the early evening and again at bedtime, when the insects are most active.
- Wash vegetables, salads, and fruit in cooled, boiled water or bottled water if there is any doubt about the local water.
- Boil water used to make up baby foods or milk.

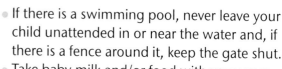

Put a sunhat on your baby whenever he is outside

Air travel

- If booking tickets for children under the age of two, ask for seats where you can use a child safety seat; airlines provide a harness for children 22–44 pounds.
- Give your baby either a feeding or a pacifier to suck as the plane ascends and descends because the change in pressure can cause earache in babies and children. Give an older child a piece of candy to suck, but make sure he does not choke on it.
- Take any food or milk that a baby needs on the plane trip. Airlines don't generally carry baby food, although they may be able to heat yours for you.
- Give your baby or child plenty to drink during the flight to prevent dehydration.

Sun protection

- Use sunscreen that protects your child from ultraviolet A rays (UVA) and ultraviolet B rays (UVB). The sun protection factor (SPF) numbers relate to UVB—choose SPF 30. A broad-spectrum sunscreen provides UVA protection. Reapply regularly, especially after he has been in water. Use a product that you know your child is not allergic to.
- Keep your baby or child's arms and legs covered as much as possible. Dress him in clothes made of closely woven fabric made of natural fibers.
- Make sure your child is protected by the shade in the middle of the day (from about 10am until 4pm).
- Put a wide-brimmed hat on your child's head that covers his neck and face and use a shade on a stroller.
- Give your child plenty to drink to prevent dehydration. If you are breastfeeding, offer your baby more feedings; give a bottlefed baby plain water.

Index

911, calling 10, 18

A
abdominal wound 51
abrasions 41
adhesive bandages 102
AED, 23
air travel 122
   pressure-change earache 100
airway
   anaphylactic shock 91
   blocked 17
   resuscitation 17
   unresponsive baby 19
   unresponsive child 22
alcohol poisoning 58
allergy 90
amputation 48
anaphylactic shock 91
animal bites 79
ankle injury 67
appendicitis 99
arm
   elbow injury 70
   injuries 70
   slings 106–7, 108
asthma 35
auto-injector 91

B
babies
   changing area safety 114
   choking 28–9
   fever 94
   hypothermia 85
   kitchen safety 112
   resuscitation 19–21
   toys and playthings 117
   unresponsiveness 19–21
back, spine injuries 63
bandages and dressings
   bandages 103
   broad-fold bandages 65

   for burns 53
   dressings 102, 104
   embedded objects in wounds 40
   hand bandages 105
   improvised dressings 103
   narrow-fold bandages 65
   roller bandages 105
   sterile pads 104
   triangular bandages 106–7
bathroom safety 116
baths, safety 116
bedroom safety 114–15
beds, safety 115
bee stings 80
berries, poisonous 58
bikes, safety 120
bites
   animal 79
   human 79
   snake 83
   tick 81
bleeding
   abdominal injury 51
   from ear 46
   internal bleeding 49
   nosebleed 45
   scalp wounds 59
   shock 36
   tooth sockets 47
   wounds 38–9
blisters 43
blood sugar levels, diabetic
   emergencies 92
body temperature 15
   fever 94
   heatstroke 89
   hypothermia 84
bones see fractures
bottle feeding 112
brachial pulse 15
brain
   concussion 60
   epileptic seizures 97
   febrile seizures 96

   meningitis 95
breathing
   anaphylactic shock 91
   asthma 35
   breath holding 32
   chest wounds 50
   choking 28–31
   croup 34
   fume inhalation 33
   hiccups 32
   resuscitating a baby 19–21
   resuscitating a child 17, 22, 24–5
   spine injuries 63
   strangulation 33
   suffocation 33
   unresponsive baby 19–21
   unresponsive child 22–7
   vital signs 14
broad-fold bandages 65
bruises 74
bunk beds 115
burns 52–7
   chemical burns 55–7
   dressings for 53
   electrical burns 54
   shock after 36

C
cabinets, safety 113, 116
calamine lotion 80
carbon monoxide safety 109
cardiopulmonary resuscitation
   see CPR
carpets, safety 111
carriages, safety 121
cars
   car seats 119
   road safety 120
   safety 119
changing areas, safety 114
checking vital signs 14–15
cheekbone injuries 62
chemical burns 55–7

eye 56
skin 55
swallowed chemicals 57
chemicals, garden safety 118
chest
   rib injuries 69
   wounds 50
chest compressions
   resuscitating a baby 20–1
   resuscitating a child 24–5
   spine injuries 63
choking 28–31
circulation
   after bandaging 105
   resuscitation 18
clothing, on fire 11
cold
   frostbite 86
   hypothermia 84–5
cold packs 74, 108
collarbone injury 76
concussion 60
conforming bandages 103
cribs, safety 114
CPR
   (cardiopulmonary resuscitation)
      babies 20–1
      children 24–5
      spine injuries 63
cramps 73
crossing the road 120
croup 34
crush injury 49
curtains, safety 111
cuts and abrasions 41

D

dehydration
   heat exhaustion 88
   vomiting and diarrhea 98
diabetic emergencies 92
diarrhea 98
doors, safety 110, 112
drawers, safety 113
dressings *see* bandages and dressings
drowning 13

drugs
   poisoning 58
   see also medication
washers and dryers, safety 113

E

ears
   bleeding from 46
   earache 100
   foreign objects in 77
   wounds 46
elbow injury 70
electricity
   burns 54
   safety 109, 111, 113
   injuries 12
   shock 12, 54
elevation slings 107
embedded objects, in wounds 40
emergencies
   action in 10
   calling 911 10, 18
   choking 28–31
   diabetes 92
   electrical injury 12
   fire 11
   seizures 96–7
   unresponsiveness 14–29
   water incident 13
epileptic seizures 97
epinephrine, Epipen 91
eyes
   chemical burns 56
   foreign objects in 76
   eyebrow and eyelid wounds 44

F

face
   cheekbone injuries 62
   jaw injuries 62
   mouth wounds 47
   nose injuries 62
fainting 93

febrile seizures 96
feet
   blisters 43
   cramp 73
   frostbite 86
   injuries 64
fever 94
   febrile seizures 96
   vital signs
fingers
   amputation 48
   frostbite 86
   jammed fingers 71
fire 11
   clothing on fire 11
   escaping from 11
   frying pan fires 11
   home safety 109
fire blankets 112
fire extinguishers 112
fireplaces, safety 111
first aid kit 102–3
   household items 108
floors, safety 110, 112
food poisoning 113
foreign objects
   in ear 77
   in eye 76
   in nose 78
   swallowed 78
   in wounds 40
fractures
   ankle 67
   arm 70
   collarbone 68
   foot 66
   hand 71
   jaw 62
   leg 64–5
   pelvis 64
   ribs 69
   skull 61
   spine 63
frostbite 86
frying pan fires 11
fume inhalation 33
furniture, safety 111

G

garages, safety 119
gas
    inhalation 33
    safety 109
gauze swabs 102

H

halls, safety 110
hands
    amputated fingers 48
    bandages 105
    frostbite 86
    hand injuries 71
    jammed fingers 71
head
    cheekbone injuries 62
    head injuries 60–1
    jaw injuries 62
    mouth wounds 47
    nose injuries 62
    scalp wounds 59
    skull fractures 61
heart massage
    babies 20–1
    children 24–5
heat exhaustion 88
heat rash 87
heaters, safety 111
heatstroke 89
hiccups 32
high-voltage (DC) current 12
highchairs, safety 112
home safety 109–19
hornet stings 86
human bites 79
hypoallergenic tape 102
hypothermia 84–5

I

immunizations
    foreign travel 122
    tetanus 42
improvised dressings 103

improvised slings 106
infected wounds 42
inhalation, fumes 33
injections, Epipen 91
insects
    in ear 77
    insect repellent 122
    stings 80
internal bleeding 49

J

jaw injuries 62
jellyfish stings 82
joints
    ankle injury 67
    elbow injury 70
    knee injury 66

K

plastic wrap, as emergency
    dressing 108
kitchens, safety 112–13
knee injury 66

L

legs
    ankle injury 67
    cramps 73
    injuries 64–5
    knee injury 66
    splints 65
limbs, amputation 48

M

marine puncture wound 82
medication
    asthma 35
    drug poisoning 58
    Epipen 91
meningitis 95
mouth
    bleeding from tooth socket 47
    burns 52

    toothache 101
    wounds 47
muscles, cramp 73

N

narrow-fold bandages 65
nose
    foreign objects in 78
    injuries 62
    nosebleeds 45

O

ovens, safety 113

P

pediatric AED usage 23
pelvic injury 64
pillowcases, as emergency
    dressings 108
plants, poisonous 58, 118
plastic bags, emergency
    dressings 108
play, safety 112, 117
playgrounds, safety 121
Poison Control Center 58
poison ivy rash 80
poisoning
    drug 58
    alcohol 58
    plants 58, 118
pressure-change earache
    100
pulse
    brachial 15
    checking 15
    radial 15

R

radial pulse 15
rashes
    heat rash 58
    meningitis 95
    poison ivy rash 80

recovery position
  babies 21
  children 26–7
refrigerators, safety 113
rescue breathing
  after drowning 13
  resuscitating a baby 19–21
  resuscitating a child 23–5
rib injuries 69
road safety 120
roller bandages 102, 105

S

safety in the home 109–19
  bathrooms 116
  bedrooms 114–15
  electricity 109
  family and living rooms 111
  fire 109
  garage and car safety 119
  gas 109
  hall and stairs 110
  kitchens 112–13
  toys and playthings 117
  yards 118
safety pins 103
scalds 52–3
scalp wounds 59
scissors 102
seizures
  epileptic 97
  febrile 96
severe bleeding 38
sheds, safety 118
sheets, as emergency dressings 108
shock 36–7
  anaphylactic 91
  electrical 12
showers, safety 116
sitting rooms, safety 111
skin
  chemical burns 55
  heat rash 87
  meningitis rash 95
  poison ivy rash 80
  sun protection 122

sunburn 87
skull fracture 61
slings 70, 106–7
  collarbone injury 68
  elevation slings 107
  hand injuries 71
  improvised slings 106
smoke detectors 109
smoke inhalation 33
snakebites 83
spinal injuries 63
splinters 75
splints, leg 65
sprains, ankle 67
stairs, safety 110
sterile dressings 102, 104
stings
  insect 80
  jellyfish 82
  marine puncture wounds 82
stomachache 99
stovetop, safety 113
strangers, talking to 121
strangulation 33
street safety 120
strollers, safety 121
stovetop, safety 113
suffocation 33
sun protection 122
sunburn 87
swallowed chemicals 57
swallowed foreign objects 78
swellings 74

T

tables, safety 113
tape, hypoallergenic 102
teeth
  bleeding from tooth socket 47
  toothache 101
telephones, in an emergency 10
temperature 15
  fever 94
  heat exhaustion 88
  heat rash 87
  heatstroke 89

hypothermia 84–5
  sunburn 87
tetanus 41, 42
throat, burns 52
tick bites 81
toes, frostbite 86
toilets, safety 116
tooth sockets, bleeding from 47
toothache 101
toys, safety 115, 117
trash cans, safety 112
travel 122
triangular bandages 106–7
tweezers 102

U

unresponsiveness 15, 16–27
  AED 23
  anaphylactic shock 91
  babies 19–21
  calling 911 18
  children 22–5
  choking 29, 31
  diabetic emergencies 92
  epileptic seizures 97
  fainting 93
  febrile seizures 96
  head injuries 60–1
  recovery position 26–7

V

vaccinations
  foreign travel 122
  tetanus 41, 42
vital signs, checking 14–15
vomiting 98

W

washers and dryers, safety 113
washcloth 108
wasp stings 80
water
  drowning 13
  incident 13

safety 118
windows, safety 115
work surfaces, safety 113
wounds
    abdominal 51
    amputation 48
    animal bites 79
    bleeding 38–9
    blisters 43

chest 50
crush injury 49
cuts and abrasions 41
ear 46
embedded objects in 40
eyebrow and eyelid 44
infected 42
marine puncture 82
mouth 47

scalp 59
splinters 75

Y

yard, safety 118

Acknowledgments

Dorling Kindersley would like to thank Phil Gamble, Anjali Sachar, and Sachin Singh for the illustrations; and Suefa Lee for editorial assisstance and indexing.

The publisher would like to thank the following for their kind permission to reproduce their photographs: (Key: a-above; b-below/bottom; c-center; f-far; l-left; r-right; t-top)
21 Lloyd Sturdy: British Red Cross br; **81** Wikipedia: CDC/ James Gathany br
All other images © Dorling Kindersley
For further information see: **www.dkimages.com**
Dorling Kindersley would like to thank:
Joe Mulligan, Head of First Aid Education, Nadine Threader, Jane Keogh, and Andrew Farrar from the British Red Cross; Cardiac Science for the loan of the pediatric AED; Hilary Bird for the index; the following for modeling:
Children Aleena Awan, Navaz Awan, Max Buckingham, Madeline Cameron, Alfie Clarke, Amy Davies, Thomas Davies, James Dow, Kyla Edwards, Austin Enil, Lia Foa, Maya Foa, Jessica Forge, Kashi Gorton, Emily Gorton, Thomas Greene, Alexander Harrison, Rupert Harrison, Ben Harrison, Jessica Harris-Voss, Hannah Headam, Jake Hutton, Rosemary Kaloki, Winnie Kaloki, Ella Kaye, Maddy Kaye, Jade Lamb, Emily Leney, Harriet Lord, Daniel Lord, Crispin Lord, Ailsa McCaughrean, Fiona Maine, Tom Maine, Kincaid Malik-White, Maija Marsh, Oliver Metcalf, Eloise Morgan, Tom Razazan, Jimmy Razazan, Georgia Ritter, Rebecca Sharples, Ben Sharples, Thomas Sharples, Ben Walker, Robyn Walker, Amy Beth Walton Evans, Hanna Warren-Green, Simon Weekes, Joseph Weir, Lily Ziegler.
Adults Shaila Awan, Claire le Bas, Joanna Benwell, Angela Cameron, Georgina Davies, Marion Davies, Sophie Dow, Tina Edwards, Rachel Fitchett, Emma Foa, Emma Forge, Caroline Greene, Susan Harrison, Victoria Harrison, Julia Harris-Voss, Roy Headam, Emma Hutton, Helga Lien Evans, Sylvie Jordan, Jane Kaloki, David Kaye, Louise Kaye, Philip Lord, Geraldine McCaughrean, Diana Maine, Brian Marsh, Jonathan Metcalf, Francoise Morgan, Juliette Norsworthy, Anna Pizzi, Hossein Razazan, Angela Sharples, John Sharples, Nadine Threader, Miranda Tunbridge, Vanessa Walker, Catherine Warren-Green, Toni Weekes, Robert Ziegler.
Makeup: Wendy Holmes, Pebbles, Geoff Portas.
Additional photography Andy Crawford, Steve Gorton, Ray Mollers, Suzannah Price, Dave Rudkin, Steve Shott, Lloyd Sturdy.

Useful telephone numbers

IN AN EMERGENCY DIAL 911 OR YOUR LOCAL EMS (medical emergencies only), FIRE DEPARTMENT, OR POLICE.

FOR MEDICAL ADVICE ON POISONING, CALL 800-222-1222.

Pediatrician

Name: _____

Address: _____

Telephone: _____

Office hours: _____

Dentist

Name: _____

Address: _____

Telephone: _____

Office hours: _____

Hospital Emergency Department

Address: _____

Telephone: _____

Pharmacy

Address: _____

Telephone: _____

Prescriptions: _____

Specialists

Name: _____

Address: _____

Telephone: _____

Name: _____

Address: _____

Telephone: _____

Police

Address: _____

Telephone: _____

Gas Emergencies

Telephone: _____

Electrical Emergencies

Telephone: _____

Notes

_____
_____
_____
_____
_____
_____
_____
_____
_____
_____